Updates in Clinical Dermatology

Updates in Clinical Dermatology aims to promote the rapid and efficient transfer of medical research into clinical practice. It is published in four volumes per year. Covering new developments and innovations in all fields of clinical dermatology, it provides the clinician with a review and summary of recent research and its implications for clinical practice. Each volume is focused on a clinically relevant topic and explains how research results impact diagnostics, treatment options and procedures as well as patient management. The reader-friendly volumes are highly structured with core messages, summaries, tables, diagrams and illustrations and are written by internationally well-known experts in the field. A volume editor supervises the authors in his/her field of expertise in order to ensure that each volume provides cutting-edge information most relevant and useful for clinical dermatologists. Contributions to the series are peer reviewed by an editorial board.

Esraa M. AlEdani • Howard I. Maibach
Editors

Nutrition and Acne Vulgaris

A Concise Guide to the Effects of Diet on Adolescent and Adult Acne

Springer

Editors
Esraa M. AlEdani
Basra Medical College
Basrah, Iraq

Howard I. Maibach
University of California - San Francisco
San Francisco, CA, USA

ISSN 2523-8884 ISSN 2523-8892 (electronic)
Updates in Clinical Dermatology
ISBN 978-3-031-83676-3 ISBN 978-3-031-83677-0 (eBook)
https://doi.org/10.1007/978-3-031-83677-0

This Springer imprint is published by the registered company Springer Nature Switzerland AG
The registered company address is: Gewerbestrasse 11, 6330 Cham, Switzerland

Preface

This collection of chapters delves into the multifaceted aspects of acne vulgaris and its contributing factors, exploring the condition through various lenses—ranging from diet and the microbiome to hormonal and lifestyle influences. The chapters aim to bridge traditional dermatology with emerging insights, offering a more comprehensive understanding of acne and its management.

The first chapter provides a detailed overview of acne vulgaris and adolescent acne, covering the pathophysiology, psychological impacts, and common treatment strategies. It sets the foundation by explaining how hormonal fluctuations, genetics, and microbial colonization contribute to acne development.

The second chapter examines the relationship between dairy consumption and acne pathogenesis. Through epidemiological studies and mechanistic insights, it discusses how milk proteins trigger insulin-like growth factor (IGF-1) signaling, promoting sebaceous activity and inflammation, thereby aggravating acne symptoms.

The third chapter explores the role of glycemic index and glycemic load in acne development. It highlights the impact of high-glycemic diets on hormonal balance, sebum production, and inflammatory pathways, emphasizing how dietary modifications can serve as effective management tools.

The fifth chapter offers an in-depth analysis of the microbiome and the potential of probiotics, prebiotics, and postbiotics in acne therapy. It showcases how these biotic interventions restore microbial balance, mitigate inflammation, and enhance skin health, presenting an innovative approach to acne treatment beyond conventional antibiotics.

The sixth chapter provides a comprehensive overview of the relationship between various vitamins, minerals, and acne vulgaris. It discusses the roles of vitamins A, D, C, E, B3, and B12, along with minerals like zinc, sulfur, and selenium, in influencing acne development and treatment. The chapter highlights the benefits of certain vitamins and minerals in reducing inflammation, sebum production, and acne severity, while also noting the potential risk of acne-exacerbating effects from high Vitamin B12 levels. Understanding the complicated interactions between these nutrients and acne vulgaris can guide more effective treatment strategies.

The seventh chapter on the skin and gut axis connects the dots between gut health and skin conditions. It emphasizes how disruptions in the gut microbiome—dysbiosis—affect skin diseases like psoriasis, eczema, and acne, underscoring the role of probiotics and diet in maintaining homeostasis between these interconnected systems.

The final chapter was to discover typical dietary patterns that have the potential to influence acne vulgaris. This was our purpose within the scope of this chapter. There are a variety of dietary elements that can have an effect on the severity of acne vulgaris, as well as the clinical pattern and comedone appearance of the condition. Fruits and vegetables, the Western diet, the Mediterranean diet, meat, fish, chocolate, and alcohol consumption are some of the elements that contribute to this condition.

Together, these chapters aim to provide clinicians, researchers, and readers with practical insights into the emerging science of acne management, encouraging the integration of dietary and microbiome-targeted therapies into dermatological practice.

Basrah, Iraq Esraa M. AlEdani
San Francisco, CA, USA Howard I. Maibach

Contents

All About Acne Vulgaris and Adolescent Acne Plus Its Mechanism

1

Esraa M. AlEdani and Yara Ashour

Contents

E. M. AlEdani (✉)
Basra Medical College, Basrah, Iraq

Y. Ashour
Al-Quds University, Gaza, Palestine
e-mail: yara.ashour98@gmail.com

E. M. AlEdani, H. I. Maibach (eds.), *Nutrition and Acne Vulgaris*, Updates in Clinical Dermatology, https://doi.org/10.1007/978-3-031-83677-0_1

1.1 Introduction to Acne Vulgaris (Overview)

1.1.1 Definition and Classification of Acne Vulgaris

1.1.1.1 What Acne Vulgaris Means?

A prevalent chronic inflammatory skin condition, acne vulgaris mostly affects the pilosebaceous unit, which includes the sebaceous glands and hair follicles. It is typified by the development of different kinds of lesions, which usually appear in regions like the face, neck, chest, back, and shoulders that have a high density of sebaceous glands [1].

1.1.1.2 Classification of Acne Lesions

There are two primary forms of acne lesions: inflammatory and non-inflammatory. Non-inflammatory lesions, known as comedones, include open comedones (blackheads) and closed comedones (whiteheads). Inflammatory lesions are further subdivided into papules, pustules, nodules, and cysts [1].

1.1.1.3 Classification Based on Severity

The number and kind of lesions present are the two main factors used to classify the severity of acne vulgaris. These factors include:

- **Mild Acne:** This type of acne is defined by a few comedones and may also include pustules or inflammatory papules.
- **Moderate Acne:** Characterized by a higher quantity of pustules and inflammatory papules as well as several comedones. There might also be a few nodules.
- **Severe Acne:** Consists of several comedones, inflammatory papules, pustules, nodules, and/or cysts (nodulocystic acne), as well as widespread skin involvement [1].

1.1.1.4 Classification Based on age

Acne vulgaris can also be classified according to the age group of onset:

- **Young Acne**: Describes acne that appears in people between the ages of 10.
- **Adolescent Acne**: This type of acne is specific to those who are between the ages of 10 and 19.
- **Adult Acne**: Refers to acne occurring in individuals older than 25 years [1].

1.1.1.5 Subtypes of Adult Acne

Adult acne is further categorized into three subtypes:

- **Persistent Acne**: Acne that starts during adolescence and continues into adulthood. This is the most common type of adult acne, accounting for 73.2% to 82% of cases.
- **Late-Onset Acne**: Acne that develops for the first time after the age of 25.
- **Relapsing Acne**: Acne that clears up but recurs in periodic attacks from youth to adulthood [2].

1.1.2 Prevalence and Demographics

One of the most common dermatological disorders in the world, acne vulgaris affects people of all ages, races, and ethnicities. It is acknowledged as the most common chronic skin disease in the US, resulting in more than five million doctor visits every year. Acne is the second most prevalent reason for dermatology referrals in the US, since it is the most common disease treated by dermatologists and the thirteenth most common condition encountered by non-dermatologists [2].

Women make up about two thirds of dermatological appointments for acne. Individuals seeking therapy for acne are typically 24 years old, while individuals older than 25 make up one-third of these consultations. Acne can occur at any age, but it is most typically seen in adolescence and early adulthood. With the peak onset usually occurring between the ages of 12 and 18. According to studies, around 90% of teenagers suffer acne, and half of those people carry the condition into adulthood. Five percent of women and one percent of males still have acne lesions at age 40.

Acne primarily affects teenagers, but it also has significant impacts on adults, especially women. According to prior studies, up to 9.3% of acne instances develop beyond the age of 25. Women are more likely to develop adult-onset acne, which is frequently linked to hormonal changes brought on by menstruation, pregnancy, or menopause [2].

1.1.3 Historical Background

Acne vulgaris has been identified and documented for a long time; the earliest records date to the time of ancient Greece and Egypt. Acne was associated with puberty by Greek physicians Aristotle and Hippocrates, who used names like varus and ionthoi to describe it. Ionthoi, in its singular form, alludes to the beginning of facial hair development, emphasizing its connection to adolescence. Similar to this, the term "aku-t," which is phonetically similar to "acne" and probably derives from it, was used to describe boils and pustules in the ancient Egyptian document known as the Ebers Papyrus.

The humoral theory, which believed that skin disorders reflected imbalances in the body's four humors—blood, phlegm, black bile, and yellow bile—evolved the understanding of acne in ancient Greek medicine. It was thought that too much melancholic blood caused acne. Sir Thomas Elyot described acne together with symptoms such as obesity and excessive urine production in the sixteenth century, and he linked acne to endocrine disruptions. Acne and hormonal changes related to menstruation and sexual activity were linked by the seventeenth century.

With the development of the microscope, significant progress was made possible. Skin pores were recognized as gland openings by Marcello Malphigi and Hermann Boerhaave, and the name "sebaceous gland" was first used by Giovanni Battista Morgagni. The discovery of the Demodex mite in tissue afflicted by acne by Karl Gustav Theodor Simon in 1842 contributed to our growing knowledge of the microbiological elements of acne.

The scientific classification and understanding of acne were significantly refined in the nineteenth century. Sebaceous gland blockage was described by Samuel Plumbe, who noted that young adults were most likely to experience it. Four forms of acne were identified by Robert Willan and Thomas Bateman: simplex, punctate, indurate, and rosacea with Rosacea has been associated with digestive problems. Early in the twentieth century, Eduard Von Jacobi rejected the idea that acne is exclusively caused by bacteria and recognized the role that seborrheic conditions play in the condition's complex character [2].

1.2 Epidemiology of Adolescent Acne

1.2.1 Age-Specific Prevalence

Most cases of acne vulgaris occur in adolescence, usually around the time that puberty begins. One of the most prevalent dermatological problems between the ages of 12 and 18 is acne, which affects about 95% of teenage boys and 85% of teenage girls. The condition peaks in prevalence during this time. Up to 50% of adults with acne still have it as adults, with 20% of teenagers suffering from moderate to severe acne.

The incidence of acne usually decreases with age, and many people report that their symptoms get better or go away as they become older. However, some people have acne well into their 20s, 30s, and even later in life [3].

1.2.2 Gender Differences

The frequency and clinical manifestation of teenage acne differ significantly between genders. Males have acne more often than females during adolescence, but as adults, the prevalence of acne reverses, with women experiencing it more frequently. Acne in men is typically more severe and manifests as inflammatory papules, pustules, and nodules. On the other hand, women are more likely to develop comedonal acne, which can vary in severity depending on hormonal swings during the menstrual cycle.

In a cross-sectional epidemiologic investigation, the prevalence of teenage acne was found to be 20.8% in females and 27.9% in boys. On the other hand, adult acne primarily affects women; 82.1% of cases of adult acne were reported in a study including 280 individuals.

The gender difference in acne prevalence is partly explained by the effects of androgens, especially testosterone, on sebaceous gland activity and sebum production. Furthermore, how men and women perceive and treat acne may be influenced by cultural and societal influences [4].

1.3 Anatomy of the Skin

1.3.1 Structure and Function of the Skin

The human skin is the largest organ, with an approximate surface area of 2 m^2 and an average adult weight of 3.6 kg. It acts as an insulating, waterproof barrier to insulate the body from the damaging effects of the environment. In addition, the skin secretes hormones, neuropeptides, and cytokines that have biological effects that are both local and systemic, in addition to antimicrobial peptides that help prevent infections.

Surface ectoderm and underlying mesenchyme give rise to the integumentary system, which comprises the skin and its appendages (hair follicles, nails, sebaceous and sweat glands). The epidermis, dermis, and hypodermis are the three layers that make up the skin. These layers serve as a crucial barrier between the body and its surroundings, protecting the body, preserving water and electrolytes, controlling body temperature, and storing fat and water. Additionally, the skin is important for the immunological and endocrine systems [4].

1.3.1.1 The Epidermis

The epidermis, the outermost layer of the skin, ranges in thickness from 0.5 mm on the eyelids to 1.5 mm on the palms and soles. It is a squamous epithelial layer that is stratified and mostly made up of melanocytes and keratinocytes. With a renewal cycle of about 2 months, the epidermis is a renewing tissue that continuously gives rise to structures like sweat glands, nails, and pilosebaceous units. Based on the location and architecture of keratinocytes, it is separated into four layers: the stratum corneum, the granular layer (stratum granulosum), the basal layer, and the stratum spinosum (also known as the prickle cell layer) [4].

1.3.1.1.1 Keratinocytes

80% of epidermal cells are keratinocytes, which originate from ectodermal tissue and go through a process known as keratinization. In order for cells to move through the epidermal layers and become corneocytes in the stratum corneum, keratin must be synthesized and degraded. These cells provide the skin its structural integrity, which makes it possible for it to act as a barrier. Skin conditions including ichthyosis and other keratodermas can result from mutations in the keratin gene [4].

1.3.1.1.2 Epithelial Stem Cells

Stem cells are essential for wound healing and ongoing cell replacement in epidermal homeostasis. Progenitor cells and epidermal stem cells are found in the basal layer. Progenitor cells divide more quickly and have a shorter lifespan than stem cells, which divide slowly and have a longer lifespan. In addition, the infundibulum, sweat glands, sebaceous glands, and hair follicles all contain different kinds of epithelial stem cells [4].

1.3.1.1.3 Basal Layer (Stratum Germinativum)

Column-shaped keratinocytes, which comprise cells carrying melanin, are adhered to the basement membrane to form the basal layer. Progenitor and stem cells essential to the integrity and regeneration of the epidermis are found in this layer [4].

1.3.1.1.4 Squamous Cell Layer (Stratum Spinosum)

The squamous cell layer contains polyhedral cells linked by desmosomes, providing mechanical strength. This layer contains lamellar granules, which are composed of lipids and enzymes necessary for the skin barrier [4].

1.3.1.1.5 Granular Layer (Stratum Granulosum)

The granular layer, which is the outermost layer of the living cells is made up of cells that include keratohyaline granules, mainly profilaggrin, which is essential for the creation of the skin barrier. The stratum corneum that lies on top of this layer determines how thick it is [4].

1.3.1.1.6 Cornified Layer (Stratum Corneum)

The stratum corneum which is essential for retaining skin pH and limiting water loss, is made up of dead cells called corneocytes that are connected by corneodesmosomes and covered in a protein-lipid barrier. Corneocytes undergo proteolytic degradation during desquamation [4].

1.3.1.1.7 Nonkeratinocyte Cells

Melanocytes

Skin pigmentation is influenced by melanin produced in melanosomes by neural crest-derived melanocytes, which then transmit the melanin to keratinocytes [4].

Langerhans Cells

Langerhans cells are dendritic antigen-presenting cells, are found in the epidermis and are involved in immunological surveillance and T-cell responses [4].

Merkel Cells

Merkel cells are mechanoreceptors in the basal layer of the skin that work with nerve endings that sense light touch. They are a component of the skin's tactile-end organs [4].

The Dermal-Epidermal Junction

The basal cell plasma membrane, lamina lucida, lamina densa, and the sublamina densa fibrillar zone make up the epidermal basement membrane, which separates the epidermis from the dermis [4].

Epidermal Appendages

The skin has different ectodermal-derived structures called adnexa or epidermal appendages in addition to the epidermis. These consist of nails, apocrine glands, eccrine ducts, and pilosebaceous units. According to some experts, skin appendages facilitate the migration of epithelial cells following injury, which in turn promotes wound healing [4].

Apocrine Glands and Eccrine Sweat Glands

Apocrine glands were the first to emerge in terms of evolution. They are only found in a few places in humans, including the ear canal (ceruminous gland), areola, axillae, mons pubis, labia, scrotum, foreskin, perianal region, and the free edge of the eyelids (Moll's gland). Eccrine glands are dispersed over the body's surface, with densities varying from 100 to 600 glands per square centimeter. They represent a later evolutionary development. People with anhidrotic ectodermal dysplasia lack eccrine glands [4].

The eccrine and apocrine glands have different embryonic beginnings. Apocrine glands originate from the same epithelial germ cells that give rise to hair follicles and initially appear during the third month of embryonic development. On the other hand, eccrine glands develop from distinct epithelial germ cells later, in the fourth month. Histologically, the excretory ducts of both gland types are devoid of myoepithelial cells and are made up of bilayered cubic cells encircled by a basement membrane. Compared to the outer layer, the inner layer cells are bigger [4].

These glands also differ in their secretion processes. Eccrine glands use a merocrine secretion mechanism in which isotonic primary sweat is expelled into an epithelial-walled duct by exocytosis, and hypotonic sweat is then produced by reabsorption of NaCl. Apocrine glands secrete in a manner known as decapitation secretion, in which the luminal part of secretory cells is pinched off and released into the secretory lumen [4].

Sato et al. (1987) described the apoeccrine gland, a unique type of gland. These glands, which are restricted to adult axillae, are said to secrete more sweat than eccrine glands. However, because there aren't enough follow-up reports, the presence of apoeccrine glands is still up for debate [4].

Hair Follicle and Sebaceous Glands

Discussed separately later.

Nails

The thin, rigid, slightly elastic structures that make up nails are made up of about 25 layers of dead, keratinized cells. The nail matrix's germinative epithelium gives rise to the permanent nail plate. Toenails grow at a pace of 1 mm/month, compared to 3 mm for fingernails. Nails protect the pulp of the finger and act as a necessary counterpressure, improving tactile perception [4].

1.3.1.2 Dermis

The dermis, a thick layer that offers structural and nutritional support, is located underneath the epidermis. The outermost layer is called the papillary dermis, and the innermost layer is called the reticular dermis. Collagen and elastic fibers, immunological cells, fibroblasts, blood and lymphatic arteries, nerves, sweat and sebaceous glands, hair roots, and some muscle fibers are all found in the dermis [5].

1.3.1.2.1 Dermal Blood and Lymphatic Vessels

In the dermis, blood and lymphatic vessels transport nutrients, control immunological responses, and eliminate waste. With capillaries and lymphatic veins spreading into the dermal papillae, they form plexuses [5].

1.3.1.2.2 Muscles

Involuntary muscles found in the skin are responsible for temperature regulation and hair erection. Examples of these muscles are the glomus bodies and arrector pili. The muscles in the face and neck are voluntary, which affects how the face and neck move [5].

1.3.1.2.3 Nerves

The sensory nerves in the skin receive the touch, temperature, discomfort, and itching. In order to maintain cutaneous homeostasis, the autonomic nervous system controls glandular secretions, pilomotor activity, and vasomotor functions [5].

1.3.1.2.4 Mast Cells

Mast cells are multifunctional immune cells in the dermis, secrete cytokines and chemokines to draw in other immune cells and are involved in both innate and adaptive immune responses [5].

1.3.1.3 Hypodermis

The hypodermis, sometimes referred to as the subcutaneous layer or superficial fascia, performs a number of vital tasks for the skin, including protecting it from injury and facilitating movement by gliding over underlying tissues. Adipocytes, which are arranged into lobules delineated by fibrous connective tissue known as septa, are the main constituents of the hypodermis. There are lymphatic, blood, and nerve vessels within these septa.

Through a variety of biological processes, such as exotrophy, deposition, and endotrophy, the subcutaneous tissue stores energy. One particular mediator of subcutaneous adipocytes that is essential to the control of glucose levels and the breakdown of fatty acids is adiponectin. The subcutaneous tissue's capacity to use the aromatase enzyme to change androstenedione into estrone further qualifies it as an endocrine organ. In addition, leptin, a hormone that controls body weight by stifling hunger and supporting energy balance, is produced by adipocytes in the hypodermis [5].

1.3.2 The Role of Sebaceous Glands

The sebaceous glands, which are found inside hair follicles, are essential to the health of the skin because they produce sebum, an oily material that lubricates and waterproofs the skin. These glands, which are located between the apocrine gland and the bulge at the level of the infundibulum, are derived from the same epidermal cells as hair follicles and apocrine glands. Lobes and a sebaceous duct make up the structural components of sebaceous glands. Every lobe is made up of clusters of sebocytes that carry out a process called holocrine secretion, in which the cell breaks down completely to release sebum, a lipid-rich material that keeps skin and hair lubricated [6].

Sebum is essential in many ways. First of all, it acts as a barrier to shield the skin from the elements, keeping it from drying out and serving as a barrier against fungal and bacterial diseases. Triglycerides, free fatty acids, wax esters, squalene, and cholesterol are among the lipids that make up sebum and contribute to its moisturizing and protecting qualities. Secondly, sebum contributes to the preservation of the pH equilibrium of the skin by generating an acidic environment that prevents the growth of pathogenic germs. Sebum also has an emollient function, which improves skin suppleness and decreases water loss [6].

Many vellus hair follicles in the face region have a high concentration of sebaceous gland acini, which makes the follicles more noticeable. The term "sebaceous follicles"describes these follicles. Hormonal variables, especially androgens, which increase sebum production, control the activity of sebaceous glands. This hormonal influence accounts for the increased production of sebum that occurs during puberty. The overproduction of sebum and consequent obstruction of hair follicles frequently result in the development of acne [6].

Sebaceous glands are involved in the skin's immunological system as well. The skin's innate immunological defense is aided by the antimicrobial peptides secreted by sebocytes, such as defensins and cathelicidins. Sebum's lipid components may also have antibacterial qualities, which strengthens the skin's barrier of defense. Sebaceous glands are essential for preserving the skin's hydration, integrity, and ability to fend off outside assaults [6].

1.3.3 Hair Follicle Anatomy

Hair follicles are complex structures derived from the epidermis and are necessary for both the growth and cycling of hair. These structures start off as epithelial buds that protrude downward, led by a collection of dermal mesenchymal cells known as the dermal papilla. Hair follicles are linked to sebum glands and the arrector pili muscles, and they are found all over the body with the exception of the palms and soles. Apocrine glands are also connected to hair follicles in regions such as the axillae [6].

The infundibulum, isthmus, suprabulbar area, and hair bulb are the four anatomical regions that make up a hair follicle. The infundibulum, which connects the sebaceous duct to the skin's surface, is a sebum-filled funnel-shaped structure. It is keratinized on the epidermis and acts as a sebum reservoir. The bulge region, which is essential for storing follicular stem cells, is located in the isthmus, which runs from the sebaceous duct to the arrector pili muscular insertion. These stem cells are essential for the growth and maintenance of hair [6].

The hair bulb, which is the enlarged lower end of the follicle that encloses the dermal papilla, is located between the isthmus and the suprabulbar area. The dermal papilla is made up of nerve fibers, cells, and a stroma rich in mucopolysaccharides as well as one capillary loop. By providing growth factors including keratinocyte growth factor, bone morphogenetic protein, insulin-like growth factor, and stem cell factor, it plays a crucial part in prompting the hair follicle to grow. These growth elements are essential for melanogenesis and the growth of hair [6].

Two types of hair shafts are produced by hair follicles: vellus hair, which is thin, weakly pigmented, and stays in the upper reticular dermis, and terminal hair, which is robust, deeply pigmented, and extends into the deep dermis or subcutis. Three concentric layers make up the construction of a hair follicle: the outermost cuticle, the intermediate cortex, and the innermost medulla. The inner root sheath is made up of three layers: Huxley's layer, Henle's layer, and the inner sheath cuticle. The cortex is made up of a single row of overlapping cells. A tricholemmal keratinization site in the isthmus zone is formed by transparent cells with a high glycogen content found in the outer root sheath [6].

Three phases comprise the cyclical process of hair formation: telogen (resting), catagen (involution), and anagen (active growth). For terminal hair, the anagen phase lasts 2–7 years, although it only lasts a few months for pubic or axillary hair. Apoptosis and the end of matrix cell mitosis are features of the catagen phase. The telogen phase, which lasts for 3–4 months, comes next. Because of its cyclical nature, hair growth and regeneration are guaranteed [6].

1.4 Pathophysiology of Acne Vulgaris

1.4.1 Overview of the Pathogenic Mechanisms

Several factors, including genetic, hormonal, microbiological, and environmental interactions, contribute to the multifactorial pathophysiology of acne vulgaris. However, as sebaceous lobules per gland are said to be greater in seborrheic acne-prone skin than in normal skin, external exposure factors by themselves are typically not able to cause acne. Increased sebum production, follicular hyperkeratinization, inflammation, and bacterial colonization are the main factors that lead to the development of acne [7].

In the pilosebaceous unit, the process began with increased sebum production, increased keratinocyte proliferation, and decreased desquamation. The keratotic plug eventually forms and blocks the pilosebaceous ducts, resulting in the formation of microcomedones as sebum and keratinocytes hold each other together.

Pathological formations known as microcomedones, which are invisible to the naked eye, develop into visible lesions. These clogged follicles will fill with lipid-rich material and produce noticeable open and closed comedones as a result of sebum accumulation and increased circulating androgen production.

Sebum acts as a growing medium for bacteria, which promotes the growth of Cutibacterium acnes (C. acnes). Lastly, C. acnes releases chemical mediators that facilitate inflammation, which spreads into the surrounding dermis by the traumatic rupture of comedones. Inflammatory papules, pustules, nodules, and cysts are the outward signs of this inflammation [7].

1.4.2 Involvement of Sebum Production

The physiology of acne is significantly impacted by the production of sebum, which is regulated by hormonal, genetic, and environmental variables. Androgens, especially testosterone and dihydrotestosterone (DHT), bind to androgen receptors in sebocytes to enhance sebaceous gland activity and increase sebum production [7].

1.4.2.1 Sebum and Acne Pathogenesis

Overproduction of sebum can cause comedones, which act as a substrate for inflammation and bacterial colonization, as well as follicular blockage. Lipids and fatty acids found in sebum contribute to tissue damage and the initiation of an inflammatory response within the pilosebaceous unit. The two primary pathogenic conditions in sebocytes are dysseborrhea and hyperseborrhea. Dysseborrhea describes alterations in the quality of sebum composition, whereas hyperseborrhea refers to an aberration in the quantity of sebum. These metabolomic alterations support the expansion and biofilm development of Candida acnes, encourage the ensuing inflammation, impair the function of the follicular barrier, and cause comedogenesis [7].

1.4.2.2 Impact of Sebum Composition

When sebum is initially secreted, it mostly consists of triglycerides, with very minor levels of cholesterol and cholesterol esters and considerable amounts of wax esters and squalene. Microbial lipase hydrolyzes the triglycerides in the secretion as it travels up the follicular canal, releasing glycerol and free fatty acids. It has been observed that 95% of the free fatty acids at the skin's surface are a result of C. acnes activity, and the bacterium generates lipase. The metabolism of C. acnes results in the production of free fatty acids, which are involved in the creation of microcomedos and inflammatory responses in acne [7].

1.4.3 Role of Androgens in Acne Development

Androgens play an essential role in acne pathogenesis by regulating sebaceous gland activity, follicular keratinization, and inflammation. The primary sources of testosterone and DHT are the gonads and adrenal glands. These hormones attach to androgen receptors on sebocytes and hair follicle epithelial cells to modify gene expression and cellular function [7].

1.4.3.1 Androgen-Induced Sebum Production

Puberty-induced increases in testosterone stimulate the production of sebum, encourage follicular hyperkeratinization, and increase the inflammatory response to bacterial colonization, all of which are factors in the development of acne. It has been demonstrated that androgen receptor blockers, such as spironolactone and cyproterone acetate, can successfully lower sebum production and improve acne symptoms in certain people.

The first cause of acne is the enlargement of sebaceous glands brought on by androgen and the excessive production of sebum that follows the holocrine rupture of mature sebocytes. The primary sebotropic hormones are androgens, androgen sensitivity is high in sebaceous glands. During adolescence, when testosterone levels rise noticeably and encourage excessive sebum secretion, acne typically starts. A microcomedo is a thin-walled cystic lesion that forms when sebum is trapped behind a keratin plug, causing follicle growth [7].

1.4.3.2 Androgen Sources and Effects

The gonads and adrenal glands produce the majority of the androgens that are in the blood. The sebaceous glands also produce testosterone through the action of several enzymes that transform the adrenal androgen precursor dehydroepiandrosterone sulfate (DHEAS) into testosterone. In the sebaceous gland, type I 5-alpha reductase subsequently converts testosterone to DHT. The sebaceous glands and the keratinocytes that line the outer root sheath of the follicular epithelium have androgen receptors, which bind DHT and testosterone and mediate the actions of androgens. Compared to testosterone, DHT binds to androgen receptors with greater affinity [7].

1.4.3.3 Clinical Observations

The significance of androgens in the development of acne is supported by clinical data. Acne can be caused by an excess of Androgen, which can arise from disorders including polycystic ovarian syndrome, congenital adrenal hyperplasia, or adrenal or ovarian tumors, even though most acne patients have normal androgen levels. Except for infantile acne, which is caused by excess androgen production by underdeveloped adrenal glands or gonads, acne usually does not appear before adrenarche, the prepubertal period in which levels of DHEAS grow. In addition, men who have androgen insensitivity do not create sebum or develop acne [7].

1.4.4 The Role of Cutibacterium Acnes

The Gram-positive bacterium Cutibacterium acnes (C. acnes), formerly known as Propionibacterium acnes, is an important factor in the pathophysiology of acne vulgaris and colonizes the pilosebaceous unit. This section explores the several processes, such as enzymatic activity, immune response activation, and biofilm formation, by which C. acnes contributes to the development of acne [7].

1.4.4.1 Enzymatic Activity

Lipases and other enzymes produced by C. acnes break down sebum triglycerides into free fatty acids. These free fatty acids can lead to tissue damage and inflammation inside the follicle, which can exacerbate acne. Because of the bacterium's lipase activity, which draws neutrophils and hydrolyzes sebum triglycerides, pro-inflammatory and keratolytic consequences result. Furthermore, extracellular matrix components are broken down by a variety of proteases secreted by C. acnes, including hyaluronate lyase, endoglycoceramidases, and neuraminidases, which promote bacterial invasion and induce inflammation [8].

1.4.4.2 Immune Response Activation

By producing pro-inflammatory cytokines and activating Toll-like receptors (TLRs) on immune cells and keratinocytes, C. acnes elicits an immunological response. Inflammatory acne lesions are created as a result of this activation, which also attracts neutrophils and other inflammatory mediators. In human sebocytes and monocytes, the bacteria also triggers the nod-like receptor P3 (NLRP3) inflammasome, which results in the production of pro-inflammatory IL-1. Moreover, TLR2 on perifollicular macrophages is bound and activated by C. acnes. This results in the production of cytokines including IL-8 and IL-12, which draw neutrophils and encourage follicular rupture [8].

1.4.4.3 Genetic and Strain Differences

The levels of C. acnes colonization in acne patients and healthy people do not differ significantly. Nonetheless, it has been noted that healthy and acne-prone skin differ in their C. acnes phylotypes. Phenotype IA strains, which are connected to acne, possess more genes associated with antibiotic resistance and are more likely to induce TH17 cells to generate pro-inflammatory cytokines such as IL-17 and

IFN-gamma. On the other hand, strains linked to healthy skin cause TH17 cells to release IL-10, which has anti-inflammatory properties. In vitro IL-17 induction may be inhibited by vitamin A and D, which may have regulatory roles in the C. acnes-induced IL-17 response [8].

1.4.4.4 Biofilm Formation

On the skin's surface, C. acnes has the ability to produce biofilms, which are complex collections of sessile microorganisms covered in extracellular polymeric substance (EPS). In addition to providing resistance to antibacterial drugs and inflammatory cells in the host, biofilms control the growth and metabolism of microbes. The genome of C. acnes contains genes linked to the manufacture of glycocalyx polymers, which promote surface adherence and biofilm development. In comparison to control samples, biofilm formation has been seen more frequently in acne samples, which may lead to antibiotic resistance and treatment failure. Because EPS restricts the movement and interaction of antibiotics with bacteria, it limits antimicrobial distribution and lowers the efficiency of antibiotics [8].

1.4.4.5 Host Inflammatory Response

Antimicrobial peptides (human beta-defensin 4 and granzyme B), inflammatory cytokines (IL-8), and matrix metalloproteinases (MMPs) 1 and 3 have all been found to be upregulated in acne-affected skin gene expression investigations. The inflammatory response in acne lesions is influenced by these factors. In skin affected by acne, human beta-defensin 2 is significantly elevated, while beta-defensin 1 is also somewhat raised. Variations in acne severity and prevalence may be related to the pathogenicity of particular C. acnes strains or the host's inflammatory response to C. acnes [8].

1.4.5 Other Bacteria and Microorganisms in Acne Development

Although the most well-known bacteria linked to acne vulgaris is C. acnes, other microbes may potentially play a role in the pathophysiology of acne. Commensal bacteria on the surface of the skin, Staphylococcus epidermidis, can colonize acne lesions and increase inflammation by releasing lipoteichoic acid and other virulence factors.

Moreover, the development of acne has been linked to fungi like Malassezia furfur and Malassezia globosa, especially in cases with pityrosporum folliculitis. These fungi create lipases and other enzymes that break down sebum triglycerides, causing the pilosebaceous unit to become inflamed and release free fatty acids [8].

1.5 Factors Contributing to Acne

Adolescent acne is caused by a number of causes, including hormone fluctuations, genetic susceptibility, environmental variables, and lifestyle decisions.

Acne susceptibility is also significantly influenced by genetic factors; research indicates a considerable familial tendency to acne. Although the actual mechanisms underlying acne development and severity are not entirely known, environmental factors such as stress, food, and exposure to particular drugs or cosmetics may influence acne development and severity [9].

1.5.1 Genetics and Hereditary Factors

Research suggests that up to 80% of the variable in acne severity can be attributable to hereditary factors, highlighting the important role that genetic predisposition plays in acne susceptibility. This section explores the evidence from twin studies, family-based research, genetic polymorphisms, and other sources regarding the hereditary and genetic aspects of acne vulgaris [9].

1.5.1.1 Genetic Factors in Acne Pathogenesis

Numerous genes, including those related to sebum production, follicular keratinization, inflammation, and immunological modulation, have been linked to the pathophysiology of acne. Although specific genetic variants linked to acne susceptibility have been found, more investigation is necessary to completely understand the underlying mechanisms. Both adult and teenage acne are frequently accompanied with a history of acne in first-degree relatives, indicating a genetic predisposition [9].

1.5.1.2 Family-Based Studies

Studies conducted on families offer strong evidence that acne has a hereditary component. The likelihood of developing acne in oneself is higher in those with a family history of the disorder. 38.8% of adult acne patients had at least one first-degree family member with acne, according to Khunger et al. Even greater incidences, ranging from 50% to 70.9%, have been recorded in other investigations. A higher likelihood of relapse in adult female acne is also indicated by a familial history of acne. In an epidemiological study involving 913 French teenagers, for example, it was discovered that the mother and father had a history of acne in the acne group (25%) and the group without acne had a history of acne (16%), respectively [9].

1.5.1.3 Twin Studies

Additional evidence supporting acne's heritable nature has come from twin research. A substantial genetic component to acne was found in a major study involving monozygotic and dizygotic twins, indicating that genetic variables are important for the onset and progression of the disorder. The significance of genetics is highlighted by the heritability of acne in twin studies, even if the precise genes and their modes of action are still poorly understood [9].

1.5.1.4 Case-Control Studies

Studies on case-control subjects have shown that those with afflicted first-degree relatives had a more than threefold increased risk of developing acne. For example, a study discovered that young people with a family history of acne had a much greater percentage of early-onset acne. In a similar vein, acne sufferers of all ages showed this tendency in another study. Additionally, a different study revealed that high school students who had a positive family history of acne were 2.3 times more likely to experience moderate to severe acne than students who did not [9].

1.5.1.5 Microscopic Evidence

Studies conducted under a microscope provide light on the genetic susceptibility to acne. Confocal microscopy analysis of adult female acne patients showed more comedones and follicles with expanded infundibulum in comparison to control subjects. This research adds more evidence to the significance of genetic variables in the pathophysiology of acne by pointing to a hereditary vulnerability to hyperseborrhea [9].

1.5.2 Hormonal Changes During Adolescence

Hormonal changes are intimately associated with the onset and worsening of acne, especially the rise in androgen throughout puberty. By attaching to androgen receptors within sebocytes, androgens like testosterone and dihydrotestosterone (DHT) boost the activity of sebaceous glands and increase the production of sebum. An important element in the adolescent pathophysiology of acne is this hormonal activity [9].

1.5.2.1 Androgens and Sebum Production

The increase in androgen levels throughout puberty has a major impact on sebaceous gland function. Increased sebum production fosters the growth of C. acnes, which in turn leads to the development of acne lesions. Androgens have a direct impact on sebocytes, causing hyperplasia and increased secretion of sebum—two important aspects of the pathophysiology of acne [9].

1.5.2.2 Influence of Insulin Resistance and PCOS

Obesity in PCOS patients can cause insulin resistance, which in turn aggravates hyperandrogenism and eventually severe acne. Free and bioavailable testosterone levels are raised in PCOS patients with insulin resistance, which further stimulates sebaceous gland activity and exacerbates acne symptoms [9].

1.5.2.3 Premenstrual Acne

Premenstrual acne is commonly linked to hormonal variations that increase the water content of the pilosebaceous unit, hence causing obstruction of the sebaceous duct orifice. Progesterone-derived oral contraceptives, which can change the hormonal balance and cause acne flare-ups, may also have an impact on this exacerbation [9].

1.5.2.4 Other Hormonal Influences

Apart from androgens, additional hormones that might affect the development of acne include insulin, insulin-like growth factor 1 (IGF-1), and adrenal steroids. These hormones affect inflammation, follicular keratinization, and sebaceous gland activity. It has been demonstrated that increased IGF-1 and insulin levels promote keratinocyte proliferation and sebaceous gland activity, which in turn aids in the development of comedones and inflammatory lesions [9].

1.5.2.5 Hormonal Contraceptives

By lowering androgen levels and sebum production, hormonal contraceptives with estrogen and progestin components have been shown to help some people with acne problems. By lessening the impact of androgens on sebaceous glands, these contraceptives can improve the severity of acne by reducing sebum production [9].

1.5.3 Dietary Factors and Their Impact

Although the actual mechanisms underlying the development and aggravation of acne vulgaris are still poorly understood, dietary factors have long been linked to the condition. According to recent research, a number of biochemical pathways, including as insulin and IGF-1 signaling, sebaceous gland activity, and inflammatory responses, may be influenced by specific meals in the etiology of acne. This section examines our current knowledge of the role that certain food ingredients have in acne [9].

1.5.3.1 High-Glycemic Index Foods

Foods with a high glycemic index (GI), such sugar and refined carbohydrates, can cause surges in insulin and insulin-like growth factor 1 (IGF-1). This surge is thought to stimulate sebaceous gland activity, increasing sebum production and contributing to the development of acne. Insulinotropic milk, dairy products and hyperglycemic carbohydrates, enhance insulin/IGF-1 signaling while lowering levels of Insulin-like Growth Factor Binding Protein 3 (IGFBP-3). By binding to the retinoid X receptor, IGFBP-3 prevents apoptosis and promotes cell proliferation, while IGF-1 decreases the nuclear levels of the metabolic forkhead box class O transcription factor 1 (FoxO1). As a result of this decrease in FoxO1, the mammalian Target of Rapamycin Complex 1 (mTORC1) is activated, promoting the hyperproliferation of sebaceous glands, lipid production, and keratinocyte hyperplasia—all of which contribute to acne [9].

1.5.3.2 Dairy Products

Because dairy products include hormones and bioactive proteins, they have been linked to the development of acne, especially skim milk. Consuming milk raises insulin and IGF-1 levels, which affect the pilosebaceous unit's follicular keratinization and inflammation. Consuming milk, especially low-fat and skim milk, has been linked to acne in several large cohort studies. For example, a study from the Nurses' Health Study, which included 47,355 women, discovered a link between the prevalence of acne and milk drinking in high school. The association between frequent milk drinking and more severe acne was confirmed by another case-control study with 358 controls and 205 patients with mild to severe acne [9].

1.5.3.3 Other Dietary Factors

Certain dietary components, like antioxidants, omega-3 fatty acids, and specific vitamins and minerals, may protect against acne by reducing oxidative stress and inflammatory pathways. To identify the precise food components that contribute to acne etiology and their possible treatment implications, more research is necessary. Acne may worsen if one consumes white bread, fatty and sugary items, and sugary beverages, according to controlled research and epidemiological evidence. On the other hand, meals like beans, salmon, and whole wheat bread may help lessen the severity of acne. According to a study by Penso et al., adult acne is currently linked to high consumption of milk, sugary drinks, and fatty and sugary items. Similarly, Karadağ et al. found that acne severity in people under 25 years old could be increased by white sugar, dairy products, ice cream, and white bread [9].

1.5.3.4 Emerging Evidence and Clinical Implications

New research points to a complicated relationship between nutrition and acne. For example, Kutlu et al. discovered that adolescents with significantly less severe acne drank more grapes, and that adolescents with significantly less severe acne ingested more tangerines. Acne in all age groups is often linked to diets such as chocolate, pizza, cola, French fries, and dry foods. On the other hand, research has demonstrated that a low glycemic load diet can considerably lower the number of acne lesions, including a 12-week randomized trial that compared low and high glycemic load diets. These results imply that dietary adjustments may help control acne, but more investigation is required to develop firm dietary recommendations for the prevention and treatment of acne [9].

1.5.4 Psychosocial Impact of Acne

Acne vulgaris can significantly contribute to psychological morbidity and, in rare instances, mortality due to suicide. Feelings of embarrassment, anxiety, and lowered self-esteem stemming from the appearance of affected skin or disfiguring scars which can negatively impact a person's social life and career prospects [9].

1.5.4.1 Effects on Self-Esteem and Body Image

Adolescence is a crucial time for identity building and social connections, and acne can have a significant impact on one's self-esteem and body image at this phase. A person's confidence and sense of worth are frequently undermined when acne lesions are visible since they can cause humiliation, shame, and self-consciousness. According to research, people who have acne are more likely to experience self-doubt about how they look and to disguise their lesions by habits like wearing a lot of makeup or avoiding social situations. These negative perceptions of oneself can last into adulthood and cause anxiety, sadness, and other mental health issues [9].

1.5.4.2 Social and Psychological Consequences

Acne-related psychological problems affect social interactions, academic achievement, and career prospects in addition to personal self-esteem issues. Adolescents with acne may experience peer rejection, bullying, and social exclusion, which can leave them feeling alone and isolated. Acne's psychological effects extend to family dynamics and interpersonal connections, as parents may find it difficult to recognize and meet their child's emotional needs. Numerous psychological problems, such as depression, suicidal thoughts, anxiety, psychosomatic symptoms, shame, embarrassment, and social inhibition, have been linked to acne in case-control and cross-sectional investigations. When acne is effectively treated, these problems often get improved [9].

1.5.4.3 Quality of Life Implications

Acne's psychosocial effects can severely decrease a person's quality of life in a number of areas, including daily tasks, social interaction, and emotional health. Anxiety brought on by acne can cause avoidance tendencies, a decrease in social interaction, and strained interpersonal relationships, all of which may impact one's quality of life in general. According to studies, people with acne frequently report feeling less satisfied with their lives and less subjectively well-off than people without acne. Furthermore, in case-control studies of young men and women, acne has been linked to unemployment. In order to address acne's complex effects on quality of life, a comprehensive approach to acne therapy must include both psychological support services and dermatological interventions targeted at reducing acne symptoms [9].

1.6 Clinical Presentation

1.6.1 Types of Acne Lesions (Comedones, Papules, Pustules, Nodules, Cysts)

Acne vulgaris can present clinically as noninflammatory comedones, inflammatory papules, pustules, and cysts. The classic feature of acne vulgaris are comedones, which are caused by keratin and sebum obstructing follicles. Which precede all other acne lesions and start off as undetectable microcomedones. The production of comedones is caused by the dilation of microcomedone follicles by the continued retention of a thick substance consisting of sebum and keratinous debris. Morphologically, two forms of comedones can be distinguished: an open comedo, also known as a blackhead, and a closed comedo, often known as a whitehead. The oxidation of keratin plugs is the cause of the black appearance.

In contrast, Inflammatory lesions develop due to the inflammatory response to bacterial colonization within the pilosebaceous unit and can manifest as papules, which are small raised erythematous lesions without pus that measure less than 0.5 cm, and pustules, which are papules with a visible collection of white pus at the surface may be tender to the touch. These lesions often enlarge, becoming firm or indurated, and are termed nodules. Cysts are a similar type of lesion with noted fluctuations. Any type of severe inflammatory acne that is not treated may leave scars behind. These lesions are typically mixed together to varying degrees in the majority of acne patients.

Comedone is the hallmark of the diagnosis of acne vulgaris—if comedone nor clinically apparent, consider alternative diagnoses. Diseases that mimic acne include rosacea, folliculitis, angiofibromas, perioral dermatitis, and keratosis pilaris. Please read (Sect. 1.7.2) part for more differential diagnosis [10].

1.6.2 Distribution Patterns on the Face and Body

Individual differences in skin type, hormone cycles, and environmental exposures can all have an impact on the distribution of acne lesions. The face, neck, chest, back, and shoulders are among the body parts with a high density of sebaceous glands where acne lesions are frequently found.

Lesions related to acne on the face usually concentrate in areas such as the chin, cheeks, forehead, and nose. The "T-zone" is a distribution pattern that denotes regions with a higher density of hair follicles and sebaceous glands. Lesions related to acne can develop on the body in the chest, back, shoulders, and upper arms, especially in those with more severe types of the disease [10].

1.7 Diagnostic Criteria

1.7.1 Clinical Evaluation and Diagnosis

Acne vulgaris is mainly diagnosed by a comprehensive clinical examination that determines the type, location, and severity of the lesions. Comedones, papules, pustules, nodules, or cysts are among the diagnostic criteria. Other skin disorders with comparable appearances must be ruled out.

Doctors usually ask about the beginning, duration, and course of acne symptoms in addition to any associated conditions including food habits, menstrual irregularities, or hormonal shifts. A thorough history of the patient should include information about the family history, symptoms, and indicators of hyperandrogenism or other endocrine problems, such as excess growth hormone or cortisol. Patients should also be questioned about using exogenous androgens, which can aggravate acne, as well as known acne-causing drugs including lithium, phenytoin, glucocorticoids, and progestin-only contraceptives [10].

To assess the extent and severity of acne lesions, a complete physical examination of the skin on the face, neck, chest, back, and shoulders is essential.

1.7.2 Differential Diagnosis for Acne-Like Lesions

During the differential diagnosis process, it is important to take into account several skin disorders that may mimic acne vulgaris. To rule out other illnesses and validate the diagnosis of acne vulgaris, a thorough patient history, physical examination, and, if necessary, laboratory testing, imaging, or a histological analysis of a skin biopsy, may be needed.

Examples of differential diagnoses include:

- **Rosacea**: A chronic inflammatory skin condition marked by flushing, erythema, telangiectasia, and inflammatory papules and pustules, mostly affecting the central face.
- **Folliculitis**: Inflammation of the hair follicles caused by viral, bacterial, or fungal infections; symptoms resemble inflammatory acne and manifest as pustules, papules, or nodules.in contrast to acne comedones are absent, and lesions are typically monomorphic.
- **Perioral Dermatitis**: A rash that appears as small red papules and pustules around the mouth, nose, and eyes; it is frequently associated with the use of toothpaste that contains fluoride or topical corticosteroids.
- **Miliaria**: A transient, papular rash that usually affect the head, neck, and upper trunk, caused by the blockage of eccrine sweat glands, typically occurring after heat exposure
- **Steroid-Induced Acne**: Acneiform eruptions caused by prolonged or excessive use of topical or systemic corticosteroids, typically presenting on the face and trunk.
- **Pseudofolliculitis Barbae**: most commonly occurred in individuals with tightly curled hair and characterized by Inflammatory papules and pustules occurring in the beard area. Short, shaved or clipped hairs curl back into the skin, causing a foreign body inflammatory reaction and potentially keloidal scarring.
- **Facial Angiofibromas Associated with Tuberous Sclerosis**: Lesions usually appearing in childhood as persistent, 1 to 3 mm, pink or red papules on the nose and medial cheeks [10].

1.7.3 Imaging and Laboratory Tests If Applicable

1.7.3.1 Laboratory Studies

The need for laboratory or radiologic tests is typically limited to patients for whom the clinical evaluation suggests underlying hyperandrogenism or other specific conditions warranting additional testing. In certain circumstances, laboratory procedures such as hormonal assays and microbiological cultures may be necessary to assess underlying hormonal imbalances or to identify certain bacterial infections that are involved in the etiology of acne. Serum testosterone, DHEAS (dehydroepiandrosterone sulfate), LH (luteinizing hormone), FSH (follicle-stimulating hormone), and estradiol levels can all be measured as part of hormonal assays to check for abnormalities. To identify bacterial species like C. acnes and Staphylococcus aureus, as well as fungal species like Malassezia furfur, microbiological cultures of acne lesions can be carried out. These cultures may be utilized to recommend the use of targeted antimicrobial therapy or supplementary treatments like oral antibiotics or isotretinoin. They can also assist guide treatment decisions, especially in situations of treatment-resistant or recurring acne [11].

1.7.3.2 Imaging Studies

The size and severity of acne lesions can be evaluated by imaging studies like dermoscopy or ultrasonography, especially in conditions of nodular or cystic acne. The extent and distribution of inflammatory lesions, as well as the existence of underlying scarring or sinus tracts, can all be usefully determined by ultrasonography.

Over the years, a number of photographic techniques have been presented to help visualize acne, grade its severity, and determine how effectively treatments work. Standard photographs are a helpful and trusted tool, but they must be processed using the same settings for illumination, camera distance from the patient, and other factors. Moreover, pictures are less reliable for non-inflammatory lesions and have limitations in differentiating between deep and active surface lesions. Acne visualization may now be optimized, and the accuracy of determining acne severity and treatment response can be enhanced with the help of modern imaging techniques.

Many benefits come with digital photography, including the ability to store a huge quantity of images with ease and the ability to analyze images automatically or under supervision. Advanced imaging methods include fluorescence photography, stereoimage optical topometer imaging (which creates three-dimensional stereoimages), and imaging with parallel and orthogonal polarizations.

The visualization of skin surface characteristics, such as papules, pore size, oiliness of the skin, and acne scars, is improved by parallel polarization imaging. Photography using orthogonal polarization, also known as cross-polarization, improves the visibility of erythema, skin brightness, and inflammatory acne lesions. It is possible to combine sebum production measurement, video microscopy, and parallel- and cross-polarized photography. Based on the formation of porphyrin and the related orange-red fluorescence intensity, C. acnes density can be seen via fluorescence photography at short wavelengths (long ultraviolet A or blue-range light).

Multispectral photographs collect visual data at particular wavelengths across the electromagnetic spectrum and identify acne using Fisher linear discriminant functions.

Clinicians can improve patient outcomes by gaining a more thorough view of acne severity and therapy response by merging various imaging and laboratory approaches [11].

1.8 Treatment Approaches

1.8.1 Topical Treatments

- **Retinoids**: Adapalene, isotretinoin, motretinide, tazarotene, tretinoin
- **Antibiotics**: Clindamycin, erythromycin
- **Other Agents**: Azelaic acid, benzoyl peroxide, salicylic acid, dapsone, sodium sulfacetamide, sulfur, triclosan, niacinamide [11]

1.8.2 Systemic Treatments

- **Retinoids**: Isotretinoin (for severe cases)
- **Antibiotics**: Azithromycin, doxycycline, erythromycin, minocycline, clindamycin, and levofloxacin
- **Hormonal Treatments**: Oral contraceptives, spironolactone
- **Other Agents**: Zinc sulfate, ibuprofen, clofazimine, systemic corticosteroids [11]

1.8.3 Physical Treatments

- Comedone extraction
- Cryoslush therapy
- Cryotherapy
- Electrocauterization
- Intralesional corticosteroids
- Optical treatments: Laser and light-based therapies, photodynamic therapy [11]

1.8.4 Complementary and Alternative Medicines (CAM)

- **Essential Oils and Extracts**: Tea tree oil, basil oil, green tea, pomegranate rind extract, copaiba oil, and rose myrtle extract
- **Herbal Remedies**: Achillea millefolium, amaranth, black cumin, chamomile, garlic, neem, turmeric, witch hazel [11]

1.8.5 Combination Therapy

- Combines topical and systemic treatments like retinoids with antibiotics or benzoyl peroxide for more effective outcomes.

These treatments aim to target the key mechanisms involved in acne pathogenesis [11].

1.9 Preventive Measures

1.9.1 Lifestyle Modifications

Lifestyle modifications can be an important part of managing acne, as they address potential contributing factors such as diet, skincare, and overall health. Here are some key lifestyle changes that can help in acne treatment:

1.9.1.1 Proper Skincare Routine

- **Gentle Cleansing**: Wash your face twice a day with a mild, non-comedogenic cleanser to remove excess oil, dirt, and makeup without over-drying the skin.

- **Avoid Over-Washing**: Over-washing or using harsh products can irritate the skin and worsen acne.
- **Moisturize**: Even acne-prone skin needs hydration. Use a lightweight, oil-free moisturizer.
- **Non-Comedogenic Products**: Choose makeup, sunscreen, and skincare products labeled "non-comedogenic," meaning they won't clog pores [12].

1.9.1.2 Healthy Diet

- **Low-Glycemic Diet**: Avoid foods that spike blood sugar (e.g. white bread, sugary snacks) as these can increase sebum production and inflammation. Opt for whole grains, fruits, vegetables, and lean proteins.
- **Limit Dairy**: Some studies suggest a possible link between dairy products and acne, particularly skim milk, due to hormones in milk.
- **Healthy Fats**: Incorporate omega-3 fatty acids (found in fish, flaxseeds, and walnuts), which can reduce inflammation.
- **Stay Hydrated**: Drinking enough water helps maintain skin health and can flush out toxins [12].

1.9.1.3 Stress Management

- **Reduce Stress**: Stress triggers the release of cortisol, which can worsen acne by increasing oil production. Managing stress through activities like yoga, meditation, exercise, or adequate sleep can help.
- **Adequate Sleep**: Aim for 7–9 h of sleep per night. Poor sleep quality can worsen skin conditions, including acne [12].

1.9.1.4 Avoid Picking or Squeezing Pimples

- **No Picking or Squeezing**: This can lead to scarring, infections, and increased inflammation [12].

1.9.1.5 Exercise Regularly

- **Regular Physical Activity**: Exercise boosts circulation, helps regulate hormones, and reduces stress, which can improve skin health. However, ensure you shower after exercise to avoid sweat buildup [12].

1.9.1.6 Avoid Touching Your Face

- **Minimize Face Contact**: Frequently touching your face can transfer bacteria and oils from your hands to your skin, increasing the risk of breakouts [12].

1.9.1.7 Sun Protection

- **Wear Sunscreen**: Sun exposure can aggravate acne and cause hyperpigmentation. Use an oil-free, non-comedogenic sunscreen daily [12].

1.9.1.8 Manage Hair and Hair Products

- **Keep Hair Clean**: Oily hair or hair products can lead to clogged pores, especially around the forehead. Try to keep hair away from your face and avoid using greasy products [12].

1.9.1.9 Quit Smoking

- Smoking can worsen acne by reducing oxygen supply to the skin and contributing to inflammation and delayed healing.

These modifications, along with medical treatments like topical creams or oral medications if necessary, can make a significant difference in acne management [12].

1.9.2 Skincare Routines for Acne-Prone Skin

A skincare routine for acne-prone skin should focus on controlling oil production, keeping pores clear, reducing inflammation, and preventing breakouts without irritating or over-drying the skin. Here's a step-by-step guide to creating an effective skincare routine:

1.9.2.1 Morning Routine

1.9.2.1.1 Step 1: Cleanser

- **Use a gentle, foaming cleanser**: Choose a cleanser formulated for acne-prone skin that contains ingredients like salicylic acid, benzoyl peroxide, or alpha hydroxy acids (AHAs) to help exfoliate and unclog pores.
- **Avoid harsh scrubs**: These can irritate the skin and worsen acne.
- **Recommended Ingredients**: Salicylic acid (exfoliates and unclogs pores), benzoyl peroxide (reduces bacteria), tea tree oil (natural antibacterial properties) [13].

1.9.2.1.2 Step 2: Toner (Optional)

- **Choose a mild, alcohol-free toner**: This helps to remove any remaining dirt or oil after cleansing. It can also restore the skin's natural pH balance.
- **Exfoliating toners**: If your skin tolerates it, use a toner with chemical exfoliants like glycolic acid or lactic acid to prevent clogged pores [13].

1.9.2.1.3 Step 3: Treatment

- **Spot Treatments**: Apply acne treatments containing benzoyl peroxide or salicylic acid directly to problem areas.
- **Prescription Treatments**: If prescribed by a dermatologist, apply topical treatments like retinoids (e.g. tretinoin) to reduce acne and prevent new breakouts by promoting cell turnover.
- **Niacinamide**: A good option for reducing inflammation and calming the skin, without causing irritation [13].

1.9.2.1.4 Step 4: Moisturizer

- **Lightweight, oil-free moisturizer**: Hydration is essential, even for acne-prone skin. Look for non-comedogenic (won't clog pores) products labeled "oil-free" or "water-based."

- **Ingredients to Look For**: Hyaluronic acid (for hydration), ceramides (to restore the skin barrier), or aloe vera (for soothing) [13].

1.9.2.1.5 Step 5: Sunscreen

- **Oil-Free, Non-Comedogenic Sunscreen**: Use broad-spectrum sunscreen with at least SPF 30 daily to protect your skin from UV rays, which can cause dark spots and worsen acne.
- **Look for Lightweight Formulas**: Gel-based or mineral sunscreens (with zinc oxide or titanium dioxide) are often better for acne-prone skin as they won't clog pores [13].

1.9.2.2 Night Routine

1.9.2.2.1 Step 1: Cleanser

- **Same as morning routine**: Use a gentle, acne-fighting cleanser to remove dirt, oil, and makeup at the end of the day [13].

1.9.2.2.2 Step 2: Toner (Optional)

- Apply a soothing or exfoliating toner, similar to the morning routine [13].

1.9.2.2.3 Step 3: Acne Treatment

- **Retinoids or Exfoliants**: Apply a retinoid product (e.g. adapalene or tretinoin) to increase cell turnover and prevent clogged pores. This step is essential for preventing new breakouts and treating existing ones.
- **Acne-Fighting Ingredients**: You can also use benzoyl peroxide or salicylic acid if your skin can tolerate them. Rotate between different treatments if needed, but be careful to avoid over-irritation [13].

1.9.2.2.4 Step 4: Moisturizer

- **Light but Hydrating**: Nighttime is a good opportunity to use a slightly richer moisturizer to hydrate the skin. Use oil-free, non-comedogenic options, and look for soothing ingredients like aloe, glycerin, or squalane.
- **Niacinamide**: Incorporating a niacinamide serum at night can help reduce inflammation and promote skin repair without irritation [13].

1.9.2.3 Weekly or Occasional Treatments

1.9.2.3.1 Clay Masks

- Use a clay mask once or twice a week to absorb excess oil and help clear clogged pores. Ingredients like kaolin or bentonite clay are great for oily, acne-prone skin [13].

1.9.2.3.2 Exfoliation

- **Chemical Exfoliants**: Use products with AHAs (like glycolic or lactic acid) or BHAs (like salicylic acid) 1–2 times a week to slough off dead skin cells, helping to prevent clogged pores.
- **Avoid physical scrubs**, which can irritate and damage acne-prone skin [13].

1.9.3 Importance of Sun Protection

When you have acne, the last thing you want to do is apply another product to your face, especially one that may clog your pores. However, wearing mineral or chemical sunscreen is crucial for protecting your skin from the sun's damaging rays, which can aggravate acne. A study published in the Annals of Dermatology journal found that using sunscreen did not aggravate acne and that sunscreen is essential for general skin health and skin damage prevention. The sun's UV radiation can irritate and damage the skin, exacerbating acne. Sun exposure can also induce hyperpigmentation, or darkening of the skin, because our skin generates more melanin to protect itself from the sun. Excess melanin production can cause post-inflammatory hyperpigmentation (PIH) after an acne eruption. Sun spots and freckles might be difficult to distinguish at times. PIH can be difficult to treat, thus it is preferable to avoid it altogether. According to recognized dermatologist Gabriella Fabbrocini, sunscreen may help prevent outbreaks by reducing inflammation and redness associated with acne. Furthermore, some acne treatments can make your skin more sensitive to the sun, emphasizing the importance of using sunscreen and protecting your skin. For example, several topical acne medicines contain retinoids, which improve your skin's sensitivity to UV light by increasing cell turnover [13].

1.10 Conclusion

1.10.1 Summary of Key Points

1. **Prevalence and Impact**:
   - Acne is a common inflammatory skin disease affecting approximately 80% of adolescents and young adults, causing significant psychological distress and potential for scarring.
2. **Pathogenesis**:
   - The disease is characterized by four main pathogenic factors: increased sebum production, irregular follicular desquamation, *Propionibacterium acnes* proliferation, and inflammation. Effective treatments target these mechanisms.
3. **Current Treatment Modalities**:
   - **Topical Treatments**: Include retinoids, antibiotics, benzoyl peroxide, and azelaic acid, primarily for mild to moderate acne.
   - **Systemic Treatments**: Options such as isotretinoin for severe acne and oral antibiotics for moderate cases.
   - **Physical Therapies**: Methods like comedone extraction, cryotherapy, and laser treatments are available.
   - **Complementary and Alternative Medicines (CAM)**: There's growing interest in natural remedies, although more research is needed to validate their effectiveness.

4. **Antibiotic Resistance**:
   - Increasing resistance of *P. acnes* to antibiotics is a significant concern, necessitating new treatment strategies and alternatives.
5. **Individualized Treatment**:
   - Management should consider individual patient factors, such as acne severity, treatment history, and psychosocial impact.
6. **Patient Education**:
   - Educating patients about realistic expectations, treatment adherence, and skincare practices is crucial for effective management.

1.10.2 Future Directions in Acne Research and Management

1. **Research on Antibiotic Alternatives**:
   - There is a need for the development of new antimicrobial agents and treatment modalities to combat antibiotic resistance in *P. acnes*.
2. **Investigation of CAM**:
   - Further studies are needed to explore the efficacy, safety, and mechanisms of action of various complementary and alternative treatments for acne.
3. **Understanding Acne Mechanisms**:
   - Ongoing research to better understand the molecular and genetic factors contributing to acne may lead to targeted therapies.
4. **Long-term Studies**:
   - More long-term clinical trials are necessary to evaluate the effectiveness and safety of existing and emerging treatments.
5. **Psychosocial Research**:
   - Investigating the psychological impacts of acne and the effectiveness of integrated approaches that address both physical and mental health needs.
6. **Combination Therapies**:
   - Continued exploration of multimodal treatments that target multiple pathogenic factors simultaneously to enhance efficacy and minimize side effects.
7. **Dietary Influences**:
   - Further research is warranted on the role of diet in acne pathogenesis to develop dietary interventions that may support traditional acne treatments.
8. **Personalized Medicine**:
   - Advances in personalized medicine could lead to customized treatment plans based on individual patient profiles, including genetics and microbiome analyses.

By addressing these key points and focusing on future directions, researchers and healthcare providers can enhance acne management strategies, improve patient outcomes, and reduce the burden of this common skin condition.

References

1. Titus S, Hodge J. Diagnosis and treatment of acne. Am Fam Physician. 2012;86(8):734–40.
2. Fox L, Csongradi C, Aucamp M, du Plessis J, Gerber M. Treatment modalities for acne. Molecules. 2016;21(8):1063. https://doi.org/10.3390/molecules21081063.
3. Schachner LA, Alexis AF, Andriessen A, Berson D, Gold M, Goldberg DJ, Hu S, Keri J, Kircik L, Woolery-Lloyd H. Insights into acne and the skin barrier: optimizing treatment regimens with ceramide-containing skincare. J Cosmet Dermatol. 2023;22(11):2902–9. https://doi.org/10.1111/jocd.15946.
4. https://coola.com/blogs/blog/does-sunscreen-help-acne#:~:text=In%20a%20study%20published%20in,health%20and%20skin%20damage%20prevention.&text=The%20sun's%20UV%20rays%20can,which%20can%20make%20acne%20worse.
5. Strauss JS, Krowchuk DP, Leyden JJ, Lucky AW, Shalita AR, Siegfried EC, Thiboutot DM, Van Voorhees AS, Beutner KA, Sieck CK, Bhushan R, American Academy of Dermatology/American Academy of Dermatology Association. Guidelines of care for acne vulgaris management. J Am Acad Dermatol. 2007;56(4):651–63. https://doi.org/10.1016/j.jaad.2006.08.048.
6. Zaenglein AL, Pathy AL, Schlosser BJ, Alikhan A, Baldwin HE, Berson DS, Bowe WP, Graber EM, Harper JC, Kang S, Keri JE, Leyden JJ, Reynolds RV, Silverberg NB, Stein Gold LF, Tollefson MM, Weiss JS, Dolan NC, Sagan AA, Stern M, Boyer KM, Bhushan R. Guidelines of care for the management of acne vulgaris. J Am Acad Dermatol. 2016;74(5):945–73.e33. https://doi.org/10.1016/j.jaad.2015.12.037. Erratum in: J Am Acad Dermatol. 2020 Jun;82(6):1576. doi: 10.1016/j.jaad.2020.02.010.
7. Moradi Tuchayi S, Makrantonaki E, Ganceviciene R, Dessinioti C, Feldman SR, Zouboulis CC. Acne vulgaris. Nat Rev Dis Primers. 2015;1:15029. https://doi.org/10.1038/nrdp.2015.29.
8. Williams HC, Dellavalle RP, Garner S. Acne vulgaris. Lancet. 2012;379:361–72. https://doi.org/10.1016/S0140.
9. Zaenglein AL. Acne vulgaris. N Engl J Med. 2018;379(14):1343–52. https://doi.org/10.1056/NEJMcp1702493.
10. Dawson AL, Dellavalle RP. Acne vulgaris. BMJ. 2013;346(7907):f2634. https://doi.org/10.1136/bmj.f2634.
11. Gebauer K. Acne in adolescents. Aust Fam Physician. 2017;46(12):892–5.
12. Kutlu Ö, Karadağ AS, Wollina U. Adult acne versus adolescent acne: a narrative review with a focus on epidemiology to treatment. An Bras Dermatol. 2023;98(1):75–83. https://doi.org/10.1016/j.abd.2022.01.006.
13. Perkins AC, Cheng CE, Hillebrand GG, Miyamoto K, Kimball AB. Comparison of the epidemiology of acne vulgaris among Caucasian, Asian, Continental Indian and African American women. J Eur Acad Dermatol Venereol. 2011;25(9):1054–60. https://doi.org/10.1111/j.1468-3083.2010.03919.x.

The Effect of Dairy Products on Acne Vulgaris

2

Madona Pakkam and Esraa M. AlEdani

Contents

2.1 Introduction

Dairy whey elevates insulin levels, while dairy casein raises insulin-like growth factor-1 levels. Both increase access to androgen receptors. This improves access to the androgen receptor for the 5 (or more) 5-reduced dihydrotestosterone precursors found in dairy, as well as supplementing the naturally occurring endogenous anabolic steroids from the gonads and adrenals [1].

The United States is a significant dairy-consuming nation. The frequency of acne in the general population, along with the "background noise' 'caused by pervasive dairy in the US diet, makes it difficult to obtain statistical significance in dietary research, It is difficult to define or create the content of dairy "servings' '. The concentration, quantity, and destiny of growth factors, growth hormones, branched chain amino acids, and anabolic steroids (and their precursors) in dairy products are

The original version of the chapter has been revised. A correction to this chapter can be found at https://doi.org/10.1007/978-3-031-83677-0_9

M. Pakkam
Department of Radiology, Mayo Clinic, Rochester, MN, USA

E. M. AlEdani (✉)
Basra Medical College, Basrah, Iraq

E. M. AlEdani, H. I. Maibach (eds.), *Nutrition and Acne Vulgaris*, Updates in Clinical Dermatology, https://doi.org/10.1007/978-3-031-83677-0_2

not well understood. This limits researchers' ability to quantify the elements that cause the follicular blockage characteristic of folliculo-occlusive disorders [1].

2.2 Epidemiology for the Relation Between Milk Consumption and Acne

A retrospective analysis of data from the Nurses Health Study II, which included 47,355 women who answered questionnaires on their high school diet and physician-diagnosed severe teenage acne, revealed a positive relationship between total milk and skim milk consumption and acne. Prospective cohort studies in the United States (Growing Up Today Study) involving 4273 teenage boys and 6094 teenage girls confirmed a link between milk consumption and acne. In the research of boys, the strongest connection was identified between skim milk consumption and acne, indicating that the protein portion of milk promotes acne. Increased insulin/IGF-I signaling is the most critical factor in acne etiology [2].

In acne patients, there is a link between increased face sebum secretion and IGF-I serum levels, whereas isotretinoin treatment, the most effective sebum suppressive anti-acne medication, lowers IGF-I serum levels. There was a favorable connection between dairy consumption and IGF-I serum levels in 2109 European women. A new systematic meta-analysis supported the link between milk consumption and IGF-I blood levels. Most impressively, the multicenter study group of the European Prospective Investigation into Cancer and Nutrition reported a substantial association between milk protein consumption and IGF-I serum levels in 4731 male and female participants [2].

2.3 Mechanism

2.3.1 Milk Consumption Elevates Postprandial Insulinemia

After a month of drinking 710 mL of UHT vitamin D-fortified whole milk daily, Mongolian children who had not previously consumed milk had a higher mean plasma level of IGF-I, IGF-I/IGFBP-3, and 75th percentile of GH levels. After 4 weeks of milk drinking, children's mean plasma IGF-I levels increased by 23.4% from 290.93 ± 93.98 to 358.34 ± 125.62 ng/mL. Fermented and nonfermented milk products produce hyperinsulinemic reactions that much surpass what would be predicted given their low GI. Despite having a low GI of 15–30, milk products have three to six times higher insulinemic indices (IIs) of 90–98. Both whole milk (GI: 42 ± 5; II: 148 ± 14) and skim milk (GI: 37 ± 9; II: 140 ± 13) had a significant and comparable dissociation between GI and II. It has already been proposed that some component in milk's protein fraction is responsible for its insulinotropic effect [2].

Skim milk has been shown to be an effective insulin secretagogue in type 2 diabetics. Except for cheese, which has an II of 45, milk and all dairy products, including yoghurt, ice cream, cottage cheese, and fermented milk products, have high insulinotropic activity. In a 1-week intervention trial of 24 prepubertal 8-year-old boys, the effect of 53 g of lean meat or skim milk (1.5 L/day) on insulin and IGF-I responses was investigated. In the skim milk group, insulin levels increased by 105% (from 22 to 45 pM) while IGF-I levels increased by 19% (from 209 to 249 ng/mL). Interestingly, neither insulin nor IGF-I levels increased significantly in the beef group [2].

2.3.2 Milk-Entero-Pituitary Axis

Acne pathogenesis appears to be linked to the enteroinsular axis. GIP is quickly released from K cells in response to glucose and whey protein stimulation. GIP is an essential incretin that increases pancreatic-cell insulin production. GIP, by binding to GIP receptors, has growth-promoting and anabolic effects on several different organ systems, including adipose tissue. Most intriguingly, GIP-Rs have been discovered in the pituitary gland, where GIP can activate GH secretion, as shown in acromegalic individuals. GIP-stimulated GH release from the pituitary may be a basic signaling mechanism for whey proteins throughout the lactation period. In fact, Mongolian children who had not previously consumed milk showed significantly increased GH levels after 1 month of intake. Thus, whey-induced GIP stimulation not only activates pancreatic insulin secretion, but it also likely promotes pituitary GH secretion, which is the strongest inducer of hepatic IGF-I synthesis. Furthermore, in dogs, GH has been demonstrated to improve the insulin secretory response to GIP [3].

2.3.3 Milk-Pituitary-Adrenal-Sebocyte Axis

GIP stimulates pituitary ACTH secretion and regulates the hypothalamus-pituitary-adrenal axis. ACTH is a ligand for the melanocortin-5 receptor that is increased in differentiated sebocytes and promotes lipogenesis. GIP-Rs are also found in the zona fasciculata reticularis of normal adrenals, and they are especially prevalent in certain kinds of adrenocortical adenomas and adrenal hyperplasia. This interaction may be important in acne pathogenesis, as increased DHEAS plasma levels are linked to prepubertal hormonal alterations and the development of acne comedonica. Furthermore, in the sebaceous follicle, DHEAS is transformed intracrinely to testosterone and the more powerful dihydrotestosterone. The activity of the converting enzyme 5-reductase is IGF-I-dependent [3].

2.3.4 Nutrigenomic Effects of Milk on FoxO1 Signaling in Acne Pathogenesis

Sebocytes and follicular keratinocytes both express the androgen receptor (AR), EGFR, FGFR2, insulin receptor, IGF-I receptor (IGFIR), and GHR. The IGF-I/IGFIR-mediated stimulation of the PI3K/Akt pathway has been found to play an important role in upregulating sterol response element binding protein-1 expression, which is related with enhanced sebaceous lipogenesis. Acne is caused by five major factors: androgen dependence, follicular retention hyperkeratosis, increased sebum production, Propionibacterium acnes colonization, and inflammatory follicular events. Puberty is a stage of transitory insulin resistance characterized by increased GH secretion and hepatic IGF-I production. Milk drinking mimics puberty-related endocrine signaling and raises plasma GH and IGF-I levels. In this sense, physiological GH/insulin/IGF-I signaling during puberty is supplemented by nonphysiological GH/insulin/IGF-I signaling caused by milk consumption, which has a powerful growth factor signaling network. The combined effect of enhanced growth factor signaling during puberty and persistent growth factor signals from a western diet high in dairy consumption eventually overstimulates nuclear FoxO1 export into the cytoplasm via PI3K/Akt pathway activation. In the absence of growth factors, nuclear FoxO1 inhibits nuclear receptors (AR, PPAR) as well as key genes and transcription factors involved in cell proliferation (cyclin D2), matrix modulation (matrix metalloproteinases), lipid biosynthesis (sterol response element binding protein-1), and inflammatory signaling (NFB). However, as growth factor signaling increases, genes and nuclear receptors involved in acne are de-repressed, resulting in increased AR-mediated signal transduction, increased cell proliferation of androgen-dependent cells, induction of sebaceous lipogenesis, upregulation of Toll-like receptor-2-dependent inflammatory cytokines, and decreased synthesis of antimicrobial peptides. In contrast, retinoids, antibiotics, and dietary intervention may raise FoxO1 nuclear concentration, normalizing elevated transcription of acne target genes that are upregulated by increased diet-mediated growth factor signaling. Various receptor-mediated growth factor signals, particularly whey proteins and carbohydrates, cause elevations in the insulin/IGF-I signal transduction pathways, which are finally integrated at the level of PI3K/Akt activation, resulting in a nuclear FoxO1 deficiency, the underlying nutrigenomic mechanism in the pathogenesis of acne [3].

2.4 The Effect of Dairy Products on Acne in Adolescence

Individuals aged 7–30 years who consumed any dairy, any milk, full-fat dairy, whole milk, low-fat/skim milk, or yogurt, regardless of amount or frequency, had a greater odds ratio for acne than those who did not consume any of these foods. When compared to no cheese consumption, there was a slightly greater chances ratio for acne. When the relationship of any milk was stratified by frequency of intake, it was discovered that consuming one glass of milk or more per day was related with a higher odds ratio for acne, although drinking two to six glasses per week was not. Stratified analyses for any dairy intake and acne fat content revealed that full-fat dairy and whole milk had lower odds ratios, whereas low-fat/skim milk had higher odds ratios than the overall summary estimates; a possible explanation for this observation is that low-fat/skim milk is consumed in larger quantities than whole milk. However, because of study heterogeneity and bias, the findings should be regarded with caution [4].

2.4.1 Results From Norwegian Longitudinal Study

The study population consisted of 2489 individuals, 1112 boys and 1377 girls, who completed the questionnaire in 2000–2001 and 2004.There were 343 teenagers with acne, resulting in an overall prevalence of 13.9% at age 18–19, 14.9% in boys and 13.1% in girls. Semi-skimmed dairy products were the most popular, with 1773 (72.3%) teenagers consuming them to some level, followed by 1264 (51.5%) full-fat dairy products and 518 (21.3%) skimmed dairy products. Acne prevalence was 11.7% in those who did not consume dairy, 13.4% in those who consumed moderate amounts, and 15.1% in those who consumed large amounts.There was a link between high total milk consumption and acne in females, with an adjusted OR of 1.80 (95% CI: 1.02–3.16).There was no connection detected in boys or in the study population as a whole [4].

When each fat variety of dairy products was evaluated independently, the prevalence of acne among adolescents who consumed a lot of full-fat dairy was 18.5%. Acne prevalence was 12.6% among those who did not consume full-fat dairy products. There was a link between high full-fat dairy consumption and acne, with a crude OR of 1.55 (95% CI: 1.03–2.31) and an adjusted OR of 1.56 (95% CI: 1.02–2.39). An connection was also discovered in girls, with a crude OR of 2.06 (95% CI: 1.07–3.97), although it was not significant in the adjusted analysis. No relationships were detected with semi-skimmed or skimmed dairy, nor with moderate consumption of any dairy product [5].

The findings support previous research that has linked milk consumption to acne. The strongest links in our study were seen between full-fat dairy products and acne. Previous research have found the opposite tendency. Adebamowo et al. published large cohort studies on acne and milk, revealing more significant connections with skimmed milk than with other types. In a case-control study of Italian adolescents, Di Landro et al. discovered a significantly stronger connection with skim milk. It has been suggested that dairy's acnegenic effect is driven by hormones and other bioactive compounds in the milk rather than its fat level. We have no idea why we only identified an association with full-fat dairy products and not with semi-skimmed or skimmed goods. It has been suggested that changing cow's milk processing procedures may modify the composition of other bioactive chemicals, as well as the anticipated change in fat content. Milk is a complex fluid comprising various proteins, carbs, and steroid hormones, all of which are likely to impact endogenic and possibly acne-promoting pathways. Cow's milk has recently attracted a lot of attention for its capacity to boost IGF-1 and insulin levels in vivo. The data show gender disparities, however associations were detected in both sexes in distinct milk categorizations. For girls, we found a link between acne and a high total dairy intake. Boys who consumed only full-fat dairy products had the strongest connection with acne. These males may have features that, in addition to or in conjunction with a high intake of full-fat dairy, make them more prone to acne than others, such as other dietary aberrations, varying levels of physical activity, or smoking. There were very few girls in this generation when compared to boys. The gender discrepancies could be attributed to differing patterns of dairy consumption in girls and boys. Girls and boys are likely to have different growth stages and hormonal influences, and they may be exposed to various environments, such as lifestyles. Adebamowo et al. note that correction for Tanner stage, a scale of physical development based on sex characteristics, in their largely comparable sample population, did not affect the relationships in either boys or girls [5].

2.4.2 Case Control Study in Kabul, Afghanistan

Numerous research in various countries have examined the relationship between dairy product consumption and acne. Eating of particular goods (whole and reduced fat milk, chocolate, potato chips, and egg), a family history of acne in first degree relatives (siblings), chicken eating, physical activity, dieting, and sleep duration were all linked to acne. Acne most commonly affects the face, which is consistent with Di Landro et al's findings. Chest and back involvement were found in 30.4% and 17.9% of the patients, respectively. We found a relationship between whole and low fat milk consumption and acne, as have prior research. However, several research revealed just a connection with low-fat milk.The link could be explained by the presence of milk-derived amino acids, which increase insulin secretion and activate hepatic insulin-like growth factor-1 (IGF-1) synthesis. IGF-1 has been shown to stimulate important components in acne etiology, including keratinocyte proliferation, sebocyte proliferation, and sebum generation. It is also confirmed that IGF-1 plasma levels are linked to acne severity. Previous research has validated the link between chocolate consumption and acne that we discovered.Our findings demonstrated a link between chip consumption and acne.We were unable to locate research that examined the relationship between potato chips and acne, although Wei et al. discovered a link between fried food and acne, while Jung et al. discovered a link with junk food.In our investigation, egg consumption was linked to acne; however, we were unable to discover papers on the subject.This relationship is assumed to be owing to the high quantities of leucine (8.5%) found in eggs. Leucine is thought to regulate lipid and protein synthesis, which increases sebaceous gland activity and plugs their ducts, respectively [5].

Previous research has confirmed the link between acne and a family history of acne among first-degree relatives (parents and siblings). However, the majority of the respondents in our study were uninformed of their parents' acne histories. We were only able to establish a link between acne and a history of acne in siblings [5].

In this study, chicken consumption and physical exercise were found to be inversely linked with acne. To our knowledge, no one has investigated the relationship between chicken eating and physical activity with acne. Further research could look into this association in diverse populations. Dieting was also found to be inversely associated with acne. Smith et al. found that following a low glycemic diet reduced the amount of acne lesions. Fresh vegetable consumption was higher in controls than in cases, although multivariate analysis revealed no link between fresh vegetable consumption and acne.

The study's strengths include a large sample size, acne assessment by a dermatologist, similar demographic features across the two groups, and data collection via face-to-face interviews. Our study had some limitations, including a case control design in which causation could not be determined and self-report of food consumption [5].

References

1. Aghasi M, et al. Dairy intake and acne development: a meta-analysis of observational studies. Clin Nutr. 2019;38(3):1067–75. https://doi.org/10.1016/j.clnu.2018.04.015.
2. Aalemi AK, Anwar I, Chen H. Dairy consumption and acne: a case control study in Kabul, Afghanistan. Clin Cosmet Investig Dermatol. 2019;12:481–7. https://doi.org/10.2147/CCID.S195191.
3. LaRosa CL, Quach KA, Koons K, Kunselman AR, Zhu J, Thiboutot DM, Zaenglein AL. Consumption of dairy in teenagers with and without acne. J Am Acad Dermatol. 2016;75(2):318–22. https://doi.org/10.1016/j.jaad.2016.04.030.
4. Ulvestad M, Bjertness E, Dalgard F, Halvorsen JA. Acne and dairy products in adolescence: results from a Norwegian longitudinal study. J Eur Acad Dermatol Venereol. 2016;31(3):530–5. https://doi.org/10.1111/jdv.13835.
5. Melnik BC. Evidence for acne-promoting effects of milk and other insulinotropic dairy products. Nestlé Nutr Inst Workshop Ser Pediatr Program. 2011;67:131–45. https://doi.org/10.1159/000325580.

Unraveling the Impact of Glycemic Index and Glycemic Load on Acne Vulgaris

3

Nereen A. Almosilhy, Ahmed M. Z. Hassan, Khulood O. Zahran, and Esraa M. AlEdani

Contents

3.1 Introduction

In the early 1980s, Jenkins et al. introduced the glycemic index (GI) concept, a system to measure the effect of carbohydrate-containing foods on blood glucose levels, based on dose-response curves from 62 common sugars and diets in healthy individuals [1]. The GI measures the incremental area under the blood glucose response curve (AUC), usually over 2 h, after consuming 50 g of a tested

N. A. Almosilhy (✉)
Department of Pharmacology and Toxicology, Faculty of Pharmacy, Tanta University, Tanta, Egypt

A. M. Z. Hassan
Faculty of Medicine, Cairo University, Giza, Egypt

K. O. Zahran
Faculty of Physical Therapy, Cairo University, Giza, Egypt

E. M. AlEdani
Basra Medical College, Basrah, Iraq

E. M. AlEdani, H. I. Maibach (eds.), *Nutrition and Acne Vulgaris*, Updates in Clinical Dermatology, https://doi.org/10.1007/978-3-031-83677-0_3

carbohydrate-containing food under standardized conditions. Then, it is expressed as a percentage of the AUC from the consumption of the same amount of a reference food, such as glucose or white bread, by the same individual on a separate day (Fig. 3.1) [1, 2]. In 1998, the World Health Organization (WHO) and the Food and Agriculture Organization of the United Nations (FAO) outlined a report on carbohydrates in human nutrition, which recommended the standardization of GI testing protocols, classifying carbohydrate-rich foods by GI, and employing GI values and food composition data in diet planning [2]. Several diets have been ranked on a GI scale from 0 to 100, with low (below 55), medium (55–69), or high GI (above 70) [3]. Fast-metabolizing carbohydrates, which rapidly raise blood glucose, have higher GI values, such as potatoes and refined grain diets. Conversely, slow-metabolizing carbohydrates, which release glucose slowly, have lower GI values, such as legumes, fruits, and vegetables [4, 5]. Moreover, GI value is influenced by several factors [6, 7], including:

- Dietary type (carbohydrate type, protein, fat, and fiber)
- Dietary form (the GI value of some fruits rises as they ripen over time)
- Cooking time (increased cooking time usually increases the GI value)
- Combining low- and high-GI foods (which lowers the total GI value)
- Individual variation (such as age, metabolism, and health)

The GI was primarily designed to help diabetics select a low-GI diet [8]. However, the concept of the glycemic index has since been expanded to include the impact of the total quantity of carbohydrates consumed. Thus, Salmeron et al. proposed the glycemic load (GL) concept in 1997, which accounts for both the type and amount of carbohydrates per serving to assess the overall glycemic effect [9]. Thus, GL represents the total glycemic response of a meal or specific diet. To calculate the glycemic load, the glycemic index value is multiplied by the amount of carbohydrates in 100 grams of the diet. A high glycemic load is more than 20, and a value less than 10 is considered a low glycemic load. Refined diets typically have a high glycemic load (mfore than 50), including table sugar, rice

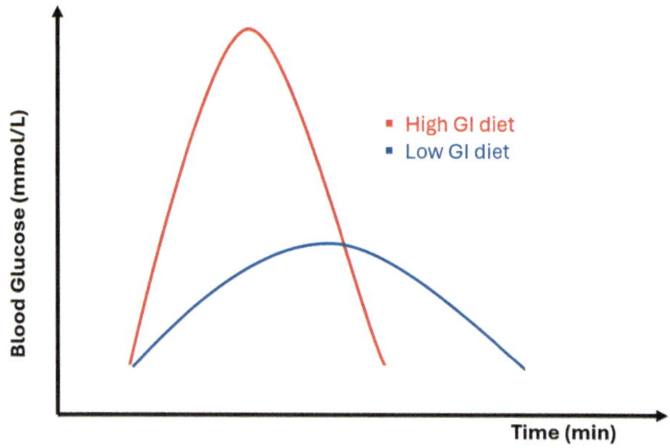

Fig. 3.1 The effect of a high glycemic index (GI) diet versus a low glycemic index (GI) diet on the blood glucose level

cakes, rice cereal, and jellybeans. In contrast, unrefined diets with a glycemic load of less than 10 are considered healthier options, such as parsnips, vegetables, and fruits [10, 11]. Notably, various dietary and cultural factors affect serving size [7]. GI is usually measured for individual foods; however, the GI and GL of mixed meals and regular diets can also be estimated [12].

Acne vulgaris is a common chronic inflammatory skin disorder characterized by the formation of papules or nodules, open or closed comedones, pustules, and even scarring on the skin. Multiple factors contribute to acne vulgaris development, including hormonal changes, inflammation, bacterial overgrowth, and genetic predispositions. Environmental conditions, stress, and certain dietary habits and medications may also exacerbate the condition. The primary causes of its occurrence include hyper-cornification in the pilosebaceous duct, increased sebum production, and abnormal microbial flora, particularly the colonization of Propionibacterium, which leads to subsequent inflammation [13].

Recent hypotheses suggest that a high GL diet increases insulin and Insulin-like Growth Factor 1 (IGF-1) signaling (IIS) while reducing insulin-like growth factor binding protein 3 (IGFBP-3) levels, leading to a state of hyperinsulinemia. Diet-induced hyperinsulinemia can trigger a series of hormonal reactions that promote sebocyte growth at the skin surface, proliferation of keratinocytes, and hyperkeratinization of hair follicles, ultimately contributing to acne formation [14, 15]. Furthermore, various studies have reported the proacnegenic effects of the Western diet due to its high levels of glucose and dairy content, which can affect hormonal levels, particularly IGF-1, as well as postprandial insulin levels [16].

3.2 The Biological Mechanisms Underlying the Exacerbation of Acne by High GI/GL Diet

3.2.1 Hyperinsulinemia and Mechanisms of IGF-1

Diets with a high GI/GL have the potential to cause hyperinsulinemia, a condition characterized by increased blood insulin levels. Hyperinsulinemia is associated with increased androgen bioavailability and elevated levels of free IGF-1. IGF-1 is essential for skin physiology as it promotes the production of sebum and the growth of keratinocytes and sebocytes. Furthermore, IGF-1 has the ability to inhibit the hepatic synthesis of sex hormone-binding globulin (SHBG), which binds to androgenic molecules and reduces their active and free forms in the circulatory system, while simultaneously promoting the production of androgens in the testes and ovaries. As a result, a feedback loop is established, amplifying the impact of androgens on cutaneous tissue. In contrast, low-glycemic-load (LGL) diets have been shown to contribute to the maintenance of higher SHBG levels and, consequently, lower amounts of free testosterone by regulating insulin levels [17–19]. Additionally, modulating IGF-1 activity also relies on its interactions with binding proteins such as IGFBP-I and IGFBP-3. In hyperinsulinemia, reduced IGFBP-3 levels and elevated IGF-1 levels can exacerbate acne by allowing more IGF-1 to bind to receptors on target tissues [18, 20–22].

3.2.2 Activation of mTORC1 and Lipogenesis

Several studies reported that a high-glycemic load (HGL) diet and dairy protein consumption increased insulin and IGF-1 signaling (IIS), reduced IGFBP-3 levels, and decreased the nuclear levels of the metabolic protein forkhead box O1 (FoxO1) [14, 23]. FoxO1 reduces androgen signaling, interacts with sebaceous lipogenesis regulatory proteins, modulates innate and adaptive immune responses, mitigates oxidative stress, and regulates the mammalian target of rapamycin complex 1 (mTORC1), a key regulator of cell growth, proliferation, and metabolic homeostasis. Therefore, FoxO1 plays a vital role in linking nutrient availability to mTORC1-regulated functions, including protein and lipid synthesis, cell growth, differentiation (such as the hyperproliferation of acroinfundibular keratinocytes), sebaceous gland enlargement, sebaceous lipogenesis, insulin resistance, and an elevated body mass index (BMI). Genetic variations that activate the signaling pathways of androgens, IGF-1, and tumor necrosis factor-alpha (TNF-α), along with leucine derived from dairy and meat, further stimulate mTORC1, thereby increasing the risk of acne vulgaris pathogenesis [23–25].

3.2.3 Glycogen Storage and Sebaceous Lipogenesis

Dietary glycemic load can impact the amount of glycogen stored in tissues, including sebaceous glands. Reducing glycogen storage through low-glycemic diets may directly affect the lipogenic activity of sebaceous glands, potentially leading to a decrease in both the quantity of lipids and the size of sebum droplets, which are major factors in the development of acne vulgaris [26].

3.2.4 Family History and Genetic Factors

It's critical to recognize that, in addition to diet, genes and family history play a significant role in the pathophysiology of acne vulgaris. Research has consistently shown a connection between acne occurrence and family history, indicating that dietary changes may be influenced by genetic predispositions [27].

Table 3.1 Summary of clinical studies on the effects of GI/GL and acne severity

Study name	Study design	Participants	Key findings
Smith et al. [28]	Observational pilot study	12 male acne patients	LGL diet group showed decreased HOMA-IR, increased IGFBP-I and IGFBP-3; HGL group showed a modest increase in HOMA-IR, and decreased SHBG levels.
Ismail et al. [29]	Case-control study	44 acne vulgaris patients and 44 controls	Higher GL diet, and increased milk and ice cream consumption positively correlated with acne vulgaris. No significant differences in BMI, body fat percentage, and other dietary intakes.
Jung et al. [37]	Cross-sectional study	783 acne patients and 502 controls	Control group consumed more vegetables and seafood; acne group consumed more junk food. HGL diet, dairy intake, fatty diet, and iodine might worsen acne.
Burris et al. [34]	Cross-sectional study	248 young adults	Correlation between dietary habits and acne severity, particularly with high-GI foods, fish, and milk. Food-aggravated acne beliefs are significantly related to acne severity.
Çerman et al. [35]	Cross-sectional study	50 acne patients and 36 controls	GI values were higher in moderate and severe acne patients; acne patients had lower serum adiponectin levels. A negative association between serum adiponectin and GI.
Smith et al. [30, 31]	RCT	43 male acne patients	LGL diet significantly reduced acne lesion counts, free androgen index, weight, and BMI; enhanced IGFBP-I and insulin sensitivity.
Smith et al. [32]	RCT	31 male acne patients	LGL diet reduced total acne lesion counts and altered the fatty acid composition of skin surface triglycerides.
Reynolds et al. [36]	RCT	58 male acne patients	No statistically significant difference in facial acne severity or insulin sensitivity between low-GI and high-GI diet groups.
Burris et al. [15]	RCT	66 acne patients	Low GI/GL diet significantly reduced serum concentrations of IGF-1.
Pavithra et al. [33]	RCT	84 acne patients	Both an LGL diet combined with topical benzoyl peroxide and the gel alone significantly reduced acne counts with no significant difference between the groups; however, only the combined LGL diet group showed significant decreases in BMI and HOMA-IR.

3.3 Clinical Trials Investigating the Relationship Between Glycemic Index/Glycemic Load and Acne Severity

Several studies have explored the associations between dietary GI/GL and acne pathogenesis and clinical symptoms (Table 3.1). An observational pilot study with 12 teenage male acne patients in a controlled feeding trial evaluated the endocrine effects of an LGL diet on acne vulgaris. For seven days, seven participants followed an LGL diet (25% protein, 45% carbohydrates) and five followed an HGL diet (15%

protein, 55% carbohydrates). On day 7, the LGL group showed a decrease in homeostasis model assessment of insulin resistance (HOMA-IR), while the HGL group exhibited a modest increase. Additionally, the study found that SHBG levels significantly decreased in the HGL group, while the LGL group exhibited significantly higher levels of IGFBP-I and IGFBP-3. These results indicate that an HGL diet may elevate sex hormones and IGF-I activity, potentially exacerbating acne. Furthermore, a case-control study examined the relationship between diet and acne severity in 88 individuals, evenly divided into acne vulgaris patients and controls. A higher GL diet, along with increased milk and ice cream consumption, was positively correlated with acne vulgaris. Nonetheless, BMI, body fat percentage, and other dietary intakes showed no significant differences between the two groups.

Smith et al. [30] conducted a 12-week randomized controlled trial (RCT) with 43 male participants with mild to moderate acne. The study compared a carbohydrate-rich control diet with an experimental low-GI diet, consisting of 25% protein, 30% fats, and 45% low-glycemic-index carbohydrates. They found that the Low-GI diet significantly reduced acne lesion counts, free androgen index, weight, and BMI, and enhanced IGFBP-I and insulin sensitivity. The findings imply an association between diet components and acne pathogenesis and indicate that nutrition-related lifestyle modifications could be effective in acne management. Another 12-week RCT by Smith et al. [28] found an LGL diet reduced acne lesion counts and altered the fatty acid composition of skin surface triglycerides in 31 male acne patients. The study suggests that desaturase enzymes play a role in sebum production and acne, highlighting the influence of diet on skin health. Additionally, Burris et al. [15] performed a 2-week RCT with 66 patients, finding that a low GI/GL diet significantly reduced serum IGF-1 levels, suggesting it may improve outcomes for acne patients.

An interesting 12-week RCT involving 84 individuals with facial acne vulgaris found that both an LGL diet combined with topical benzoyl peroxide 2.5% gel and the gel alone significantly reduced acne counts, with no significant difference between the groups, likely due to the use of the benzoyl peroxide gel in both treatments. Nevertheless, differences in BMI and HOMA-IR between the groups were statistically significant. The group that adhered to the LGL diet showed decreases in both BMI and HOMA-IR values, whereas the group that only used benzoyl peroxide gel did not observe such reductions.

In a cross-sectional study of 248 young adults in New York City, participants completed questionnaires on acne severity, dietary habits, acne-specific quality of life, food-aggravated acne beliefs, demographics, and anthropometric data. The study showed a correlation between dietary habits and acne severity, particularly with high-GI foods, fish, and milk. Food-aggravated acne beliefs were significantly related to acne severity. Another Turkish cross-sectional study of 50 acne vulgaris patients and 36 health controls examined the relationships between dietary GI/GL, acne severity, and adiponectin levels. GI results were significantly higher in moderate and severe acne patients than in those with mild acne, indicating a positive correlation with disease severity. Moreover, acne patients had significantly lower serum adiponectin levels compared to controls, with a negative association between adiponectin and glycemic index, suggesting that low GI diets may reduce acne severity by improving metabolic and immune functions.

On the other hand, an Australian study of 58 adolescent males found no significant difference in facial acne severity or insulin sensitivity between low-GI and high-GI diet groups over 8 weeks. However, the study's short duration and assessment methods may have limited the findings, suggesting that longer trials with more sensitive tools are needed.

A Korean study evaluated dietary intake and its association with acne vulgaris, including 783 patients with acne and 502 controls. The study demonstrated that the control group had a higher intake of vegetables (green, yellow leafy, cruciferous) and seafood (bluefin tuna, oily fish, white fish) compared to the acne group. Meanwhile, patients with acne consumed more junk food, snacks, fried and instant noodles, carbonated drinks, stewed chicken, nuts, seaweed, braised and roast pork, and processed cheeses. Acne patients also often skipped breakfast and had less regular meal intervals than the control group. The study also found sexual differences in IGF-1 and IGFBP-3 levels. Findings concluded that an HGL diet, dairy intake, a fatty diet, iodine in the Korean diet, and inconsistent dietary habits were shown to exacerbate acne symptoms.

As previously elaborated, various trials have shown controversial results, which align with a recent systematic review that also revealed conflicting evidence in studies examining the link between diet and acne severity. The review highlighted that, while the connection between diet and acne pathogenesis is weak, it is significantly influenced by high GI/GL and carbohydrate intake. In certain populations, especially those following a Western diet, increased dairy consumption may trigger acne pathogenesis. Additionally, the review suggests that the impact of diet on acne may be influenced by factors such as sex and ethnicity.

References

1. Jenkins DJ, Wolever TM, Taylor RH, Barker H, Fielden H, Baldwin JM, et al. Glycemic index of foods: a physiological basis for carbohydrate exchange. Am J Clin Nutr. 1981;34(3):362–6.
2. Joint FAO. Carbohydrates in human nutrition. FAO; 1998.
3. Brand-Miller J, Foster-Powell K, Holt S. The new glucose revolution complete guide to glycemic index values. Da Capo Lifelong; 2003.
4. Kim D. Glycemic index. In: Obesity. Elsevier; 2020. p. 183–9.
5. Brouns F, Bjorck I, Frayn KN, Gibbs AL, Lang V, Slama G, et al. Glycaemic index methodology. Nutr Res Rev. 2005;18(1):145–71.
6. Björck I, Granfeldt Y, Liljeberg H, Tovar J, Asp NG. Food properties affecting the digestion and absorption of carbohydrates. Am J Clin Nutr. 1994;59(3 Suppl):699S–705S.
7. Rakel D, Onna LM. Glycemic index and glycemic load. In: Rakel D, editor. Integrative medicine. 3rd ed. Elsevier; 2018. p. 863–868.e1. Chapter 87. https://d2ogjlfjkptkow.cloudfront.net/putextbook/38905.pdf.
8. Jenkins DJ, Wolever TM, Jenkins AL, Thorne MJ, Lee R, Kalmusky J, et al. The glycaemic index of foods tested in diabetic patients: a new basis for carbohydrate exchange favouring the use of legumes. Diabetologia. 1983;24(4):257–64.

9. Salmerón J, Manson JE, Stampfer MJ, Colditz GA, Wing AL, Willett WC. Dietary fiber, glycemic load, and risk of non-insulin-dependent diabetes mellitus in women. JAMA. 1997;277(6):472–7.
10. Suh DH, editor. Acne: current concepts and management. Cham: Springer International Publishing; 2021.
11. Salmerón J, Ascherio A, Rimm EB, Colditz GA, Spiegelman D, Jenkins DJ, et al. Dietary fiber, glycemic load, and risk of NIDDM in men. Diabetes Care. 1997;20(4):545–50.
12. Wolever TM, Jenkins DJ. The use of the glycemic index in predicting the blood glucose response to mixed meals. Am J Clin Nutr. 1986;43(1):167–72.
13. Baldwin H, Tan J. Effects of diet on acne and its response to treatment. Am J Clin Dermatol. 2021;22(1):55–65.
14. Berra B, Rizzo AM. Glycemic index, glycemic load: new evidence for a link with acne. J Am Coll Nutr. 2009;28(Suppl):450S–4S.
15. Burris J, Shikany JM, Rietkerk W, Woolf K. A low glycemic index and glycemic load diet decreases insulin-like growth factor-1 among adults with moderate and severe acne: a short-duration, 2-week randomized controlled trial. J Acad Nutr Diet. 2018;118(10):1874–85.
16. Meixiong J, Ricco C, Vasavda C, Ho BK. Diet and acne: a systematic review. JAAD Int. 2022;7:95–112.
17. Singh A, Hamilton-Fairley D, Koistinen R, Seppälä M, James VH, Franks S, et al. Effect of insulin-like growth factor-type I (IGF-I) and insulin on the secretion of sex hormone binding globulin and IGF-I binding protein (IBP-I) by human hepatoma cells. J Endocrinol. 1990;124(2):R1–3.
18. Brismar K, Fernqvist-Forbes E, Wahren J, Hall K. Effect of insulin on the hepatic production of insulin-like growth factor-binding protein-1 (IGFBP-1), IGFBP-3, and IGF-I in insulin-dependent diabetes. J Clin Endocrinol Metab. 1994;79(3):872–8.
19. Plymate SR, Matej LA, Jones RE, Friedl KE. Inhibition of sex hormone-binding globulin production in the human hepatoma (Hep G2) cell line by insulin and prolactin. J Clin Endocrinol Metab. 1988;67(3):460–4.
20. Cordain L, Eades MR, Eades MD. Hyperinsulinemic diseases of civilization: more than just syndrome X. Comp Biochem Physiol A Mol Integr Physiol. 2003;136(1):95–112.
21. Crave JC, Lejeune H, Brébant C, Baret C, Pugeat M. Differential effects of insulin and insulin-like growth factor I on the production of plasma steroid-binding globulins by human hepatoblastoma-derived (Hep G2) cells. J Clin Endocrinol Metab. 1995;80(4):1283–9.
22. Cordain L, Lindeberg S, Hurtado M, Hill K, Eaton SB, Brand-Miller J. Acne vulgaris: a disease of Western civilization. Arch Dermatol. 2002;138(12):1584–90.
23. Melnik BC, Zouboulis CC. Potential role of F ox O 1 and m TORC 1 in the pathogenesis of W estern diet-induced acne. Exp Dermatol. 2013;22(5):311–5.
24. Mirdamadi Y, Bommhardt U, Goihl A, Guttek K, Zouboulis CC, Quist S, et al. Insulin and Insulin-like growth factor-1 can activate the phosphoinositide-3-kinase/Akt/FoxO1 pathway in T cells in vitro. Dermatoendocrinol. 2017;9(1):e1356518.
25. Agamia NF, Abdallah DM, Sorour O, Mourad B, Younan DN. Skin expression of mammalian target of rapamycin and forkhead box transcription factor O1, and serum insulin-like growth factor-1 in patients with acne vulgaris and their relationship with diet. Br J Dermatol. 2016;174(6):1299–307.
26. Kiens B, Richter EA. Types of carbohydrate in an ordinary diet affect insulin action and muscle substrates in humans. Am J Clin Nutr. 1996;63(1):47–53.
27. Heng AHS, Chew FT. Systematic review of the epidemiology of acne vulgaris. Sci Rep. 2020;10(1):5754.
28. Smith R, Mann N, Mäkeläinen H, Roper J, Braue A, Varigos G. A pilot study to determine the short-term effects of a low glycemic load diet on hormonal markers of acne: a nonrandomized, parallel, controlled feeding trial. Mol Nutr Food Res. 2008;52(6):718–26.
29. Ismail NH, Manaf ZA, Azizan NZ. High glycemic load diet, milk and ice cream consumption are related to acne vulgaris in Malaysian young adults: a case control study. BMC Dermatol. 2012;12:13.

30. Smith RN, Mann NJ, Braue A, Mäkeläinen H, Varigos GA. A low-glycemic-load diet improves symptoms in acne vulgaris patients: a randomized controlled trial. Am J Clin Nutr. 2007;86(1):107–15.
31. Smith RN, Mann NJ, Braue A, Mäkeläinen H, Varigos GA. The effect of a high-protein, low glycemic-load diet versus a conventional, high glycemic-load diet on biochemical parameters associated with acne vulgaris: a randomized, investigator-masked, controlled trial. J Am Acad Dermatol. 2007;57(2):247–56.
32. Smith RN, Braue A, Varigos GA, Mann NJ. The effect of a low glycemic load diet on acne vulgaris and the fatty acid composition of skin surface triglycerides. J Dermatol Sci. 2008;50(1):41–52.
33. Pavithra G, Upadya GM, Rukmini MS. A randomized controlled trial of topical benzoyl peroxide 2.5% gel with a low glycemic load diet versus topical benzoyl peroxide 2.5% gel with a normal diet in acne (grades 1–3). Indian J Dermatol Venereol Leprol. 2019;85(5):486–90.
34. Burris J, Rietkerk W, Woolf K. Relationships of self-reported dietary factors and perceived acne severity in a cohort of New York young adults. J Acad Nutr Diet. 2014;114(3):384–92.
35. Çerman AA, Aktaş E, Altunay İK, Arıcı JE, Tulunay A, Ozturk FY. Dietary glycemic factors, insulin resistance, and adiponectin levels in acne vulgaris. J Am Acad Dermatol. 2016;75(1):155–62.
36. Reynolds RC, Lee S, Choi JYJ, Atkinson FS, Stockmann KS, Petocz P, et al. Effect of the glycemic index of carbohydrates on acne vulgaris. Nutrients. 2010;2(10):1060–72.
37. Jung JY, Yoon MY, Min SU, Hong JS, Choi YS, Suh DH. The influence of dietary patterns on acne vulgaris in Koreans. Eur J Dermatol. 2010;20(6):768–72.

The Effect of Fats on Acne Vulgaris

4

Rama Jamal Eddin Haboush, Mohamed Abdalla Rashed,
and Esraa M. AlEdani

Contents

4.1 Introduction to the Main Types of Fats and Their Effects on Acne

There are different types of fats in our diet, and to understand their effect on acne we should differentiate between them:

1. Saturated Fatty Acids (SFA), whose main sources are meat, dairy products, and hard fats and oils such as butter, lard, and palm oil.
2. Trans fats, which are partially hydrogenated plant oils in baked and fried foods.
3. Polyunsaturated Fatty Acids (PUFAs) e.g. Omega-3 and Omega-6, it is present in Many plants and plant oils, oily fish, seeds, and nuts [1].

R. J. E. Haboush (✉)
Faculty of Pharmacy, Cairo University, Giza, Egypt

M. A. Rashed
Faculty of Medicine, Al-Azhar University, Cairo, Egypt

E. M. AlEdani
Basra Medical College, Basrah, Iraq

E. M. AlEdani, H. I. Maibach (eds.), *Nutrition and Acne Vulgaris*, Updates in Clinical Dermatology, https://doi.org/10.1007/978-3-031-83677-0_4

World Health Organization (WHO) Dietary fat advice focuses on reducing the intake of unhealthy Saturated and trans-fatty acids to 10% and 1%—respectively—or less of total energy intake and replacing them with unsaturated fatty acids [2].

The incidence of the studies that focus on fats' correlation with Acne vulgaris increases over time and the recent evidence reveals that dietary fats play a role in acne and its treatment.

Studies showed that the Western diet—which contains high levels of saturated fatty acids (SFA)—plays a vital role in Comidogensis and promotes metabolic alterations like activating mammalian target of rapamycin complex 1 (mTORC1) the anabolism and lipogenesis regulator and as a sequence increasing the levels of the transcription factors peroxisome proliferator-activated receptor-γ (PPARγ) and sterol response element binding protein-1c (SREBP-1c) which promote sebum production and inflammatory Acne vulgaris [3]. Also, Numerous worldwide Observations have found a positive significant correlation between dietary saturated/trans fats and acne vulgaris [4–14]. On the other hand, multiple studies demonstrated the ability of omega-3 to ameliorate acne and to reduce sebum production due to inhibiting mTORC1, and SREBP-1c [15, 16].

Additionally, it inhibits acne inflammatory mediators [17–21]. While omega-6 compounds are linked to the production of inflammatory mediators [22].

4.2 The Role of Saturated and Trans-fats in Acne Vulgaris and Inflammation

Acne vulgaris is closely associated with the Western diet because it contains high levels of saturated fatty acids (SFA) and low levels of polyunsaturated fatty acids (PUFAs) [3].

Western diet is well known for its high content of SFA, and palmitic acid is the predominant SFA in this diet. Palmitic acid accounts for approximately 30% of total fatty acids in the human body [23, 24]. Palmitic acid can be found in different concentrations in some vegetable oils and animal products like meat—with a higher percentage in processed meat—and dairy products [25].

Increased dietary palmitate consumption leads to metabolic alterations promoting sebofolicular inflammasomopathy Acne vulgaris. High levels of palmitate activate the serine/threonine kinase mammalian target of rapamycin complex 1 (mTORC1) the anabolism and lipogenesis regulator and that leads to increased levels of the (PPARγ) and SREBP-1c which promote sebum production. These metabolic alterations lead to hyperseborrhea and dyssrborrhea resulting in a high follicular level of free palmitate and oleate that promotes comedogensis and inflammation as well as keratinocyte proliferation.

Dietary recommendations include restricting products that promote acne, such as SFA and trans fats. Studies showed that a paleolithic diet—vegetables and fish—is a promising nutrition therapy for acne vulgaris as it is rich in ω3-fatty acids which decreases mTORc1 activation [3].

4.2.1 Dietary Fats and Insulin and Its Relationship with Acne Vulgaris

It is well known that the primary factor that triggers insulin production is Glucose but, fatty acids are also one of the factors that stimulate insulin production.

Insulin production stimulates the phosphatidylinositide-3-kinase (PI3K) pathway which generates multiple effects in different tissues and organs leading to acne development, some common effects are:

1. Mediates sebaceous lipogenesis and cell growth by decreasing the metabolic transcription factor forkhead box O1 (FoxO1) the negative regulator of the transcriptional factors; liver X receptor-α, androgen receptor, (PPARγ) and (SREBP-1c) [3, 25].
2. Causes lipid accumulation in sebocyte, and upregulation of the inflammatory mediators. By Activating hypoxia-inducible factor 1a (HIF-1a).
3. Increases the inflammation and lipid synthesis by activating mTORC1 [25].

4.2.2 Worldwide Observational Studies Evaluation on the Link Between Acne and Dietary Fat Pattern

Numerous worldwide observations have been conducted in the last decade to examine the relationship between dietary fats—as a trigger—and Acne. All these studies have unequivocally revealed a significant correlation between dietary saturated/trans fats and acne vulgaris [4–14]. Also, Burries et al. reported that frequent consumption of fatty foods alongside low consumption of raw vegetables, fruits, and fish—protective agents against acne—is considered an aggravating factor for Acne [5].

4.3 Introduction to PUFAs and Essential Fatty Acids

Polyunsaturated fatty acids (PUFAs) are defined as fatty acids with more than one double bond in their structure. They exert their beneficial effect primarily through omega-3 and omega-6 and can be classified as either essential or conditionally essential according to the body's ability to synthesize them [26]. Essential fatty acids (EFAs) such as linoleic acid (LA) and α-linolenic acid (ALA) cannot be synthesized by the body thus must be obtained from food, whereas conditionally EFAs such as eicosapentaenoic acid (EPA), γ-linolenic acid (GLA), arachidonic (ARA) and docosahexaenoic acid (DHA) are synthesized in insufficient amount from the conversion of the EFAs, emphasizing the importance of consuming both of them in diet to meet the physiological body needs [27].

4.3.1 Metabolism of Omega-3 and Omega-6 Fatty Acids

Omega-3 fatty acids are commonly found in fatty fish such as salmon and mackerel and plant-based sources like flaxseeds. On the other hand, omega-6 fatty acids are prevalent in animal products like eggs and poultry, as well as in plant oils such as corn, safflower, and soybean oil [27]. Being metabolized to various lipid mediators, they further participate in the progression or prevention of many diseases. While omega-6 compounds are linked to the production of inflammatory mediators, omega-3 compounds are thought to have an opposing or natural effect [28]. The metabolism of PUFAs ends with the generation of specialized pro-resolving mediators (SPMs) or inflammatory mediators based on the substrate and the condition [22, 29]. For example, the oxidation of ARA, an omega-6 compound ends up with a set of compounds such as prostaglandins (e.g. PGD2, PGE2, PGF2), prostacyclin (PGI2), or thromboxane TXA2 expressing a protective or inflammatory properties according to the end product [22, 30].

4.3.2 Role of PUFAs in Acne Vulgaris and Inflammation

Omega-3 can hinder the inflammatory sequence of this cascade by competing with ARA and thus reducing ARA inflammatory mediators specifically interleukin 4, prostaglandin E2 (PGE2) and thromboxane A2 and elevating thromboxane A3, prostacyclin (PGI3), leukotriene B5, a weaker inducers of inflammation [17–21]. The same metabolism process happens with EPA and DHA, omega-3 compounds with a key difference in the cascade end by having anti-inflammatory mediators upon the action of lipoxygenase like resolvins and protectins [31]. Acne comes in contact with PUFAs because they have a substantial effect on skin health [22]. While omega-6 prostaglandins at low concentrations are part of the skin's physiological process, they can cause inflammatory reactions at high concentrations [32].

Lately, (mTORC1) which is a sensor of the cell's nutritional status has been linked to diet-induced acne through the proliferation of sebocytes. The cells that produce sebum provide the favored environment for *Propionibacterium acnes* overgrowth. Hence the ability of omega-3 to inhibit mTORC1 can be used to ameliorate acne [15, 16]. Additionally, omega-3 inhibits SREBP-1c, a protein that plays a key role in regulating the production of fatty acids and that leads also to decreased sebum production and prevents sebaceous glands obstruction [3]. Omega-3 is also thought to influence negatively different inflammatory cells including monocytes, t-cells, and circulating granulocytes [33, 34]. Additionally, it inhibits IL-1, IL6, IL-8, and TNF-α secretion, a main acne development mediator [19, 35, 36].

Multiple studies have been conducted to evaluate the effects of PUFAs on acne, Jung et al. performed a randomized double-blind controlled trial investigating the influence of omega-3 (EPA and DHA) and omega-6 (GLA) on a group of adolescents having mild to moderate acne and compare it with a control group with no intervention. They found a significant reduction in acne and non-acne inflammatory lesions demonstrated by Hematoxylin & eosin staining after 10 weeks of intervention [37]. Also, an observational trial tracked five cases of self-administrated omega-3 over 2 months and found a significant reduction in the total inflammatory papules count [20]. In addition to that, an old epidemiological study concluded that adolescents who eat large amounts of omega-3-rich food are less likely to have acne vulgaris and that it may have a beneficial effect as well [38].

Finally, omega-6 to omega-3 ratio is typically much higher in westernized rather than non-westernized food [39]. Balancing this ratio is crucial for preventing acne development and before that maintaining the overall body health [19, 40].

References

1. Mayo Clinic. Dietary fat: know which to choose. 2023.; https://www.mayoclinic.org/healthy-lifestyle/nutrition-and-healthy-eating/in-depth/fat/art-20045550.
2. World Health Organization. Saturated fatty acid and trans-fatty acid intake for adults and children: WHO guideline. 2023.; https://www.who.int/publications/i/item/9789240073630.
3. Melnik BC. Linking diet to acne metabolomics, inflammation, and comedogenesis: an update. Clin Cosmet Investig Dermatol. 2015;8:371–88.
4. Dall'Oglio F, Nasca MR, Fiorentini F, Micali G. Diet and acne: review of the evidence from 2009 to 2020. Int J Dermatol. 2021;60(6):672–85.
5. Burris J, Rietkerk W, Woolf K. Relationships of self-reported dietary factors and perceived acne severity in a cohort of New York young adults. J Acad Nutr Diet. 2014;114:384–92.
6. Wei B, Pang Y, Zhu H, et al. The epidemiology of adolescent acne in North East China. J Eur Acad Dermatol Venereol. 2010;24:953–7.
7. Jung JY, Yoon MY, Min SU, et al. The influence of dietary patterns on acne vulgaris in Koreans. Eur J Dermatol. 2010;20:768–72.
8. Aksu AE, Metintas S, Saracoglu ZN, et al. Acne: prevalence and relationship with dietary habits in Eskisehir, Turkey. J EurAcad Dermatol Venereol. 2012;26:1503–9.
9. Abo El-Fetoh NM, Alenezi NG, Alshamari NG, et al. Epidemiology of acne vulgaris in adolescent male students in Arar, Kingdom of Saudi Arabia. J Egypt Public Health Assoc. 2016;91:144–9.
10. Alkhabbaz M, Al-Taiar A, Saeed M, et al. Predictors of acne vulgaris among adolescents in Kuwait. Med Princ Pract. 2020;29:310–7.
11. Kaushik M, Gupta S, Mahendra A. Living with acne: belief and perception in a sample of Indian youths. Indian J Dermatol. 2017;62:491–7.
12. George RM, Sridharan R. Factors aggravating or precipitating acne in Indian adults: a hospital-based study of 110 cases. Indian J Dermatol. 2018;63:328–31.
13. Guertler A, Volsky A, Eijkenboom Q, Fiedler T, French LE, Reinholz M. Dietary patterns in acne and rosacea patients—a controlled study and comprehensive analysis. Nutrients. 2023;15(20):4405.
14. Khoirunnisa S, Intiyati A, Hatijah N. The relationship between carbohydrate and saturated fat intake with acne vulgaris in grade 3 female students at Department of Nutrition Poltekkes Kemenkes Surabaya. J Nutr Explor. 2023;1(1):29–39.
15. Melnik BC, Zouboulis CC. Potential role of FoxO1 and mTORC1 in the pathogenesis of Western diet-induced acne. Exp Dermatol. 2013;22(5):311–5.
16. Melnik B. The role of mTORC1 in acne pathogenesis and treatment. Exp Rev Dermatol. 2014;8(6):617–22. https://doi.org/10.1586/17469872.2013.846514.
17. Eriksen BB, Kåre DL. Open trial of supplements of omega 3 and 6 fatty acids, vitamins and minerals in atopic dermatitis. J Dermatolog Treat. 2006;17(2):82–5.
18. Logan AC. Omega-3 fatty acids and acne. Arch Dermatol. 2003;139(7):941–2; author reply 942–943.
19. Simopoulos AP. Omega-3 fatty acids in inflammation andautoimmune diseases. J Am Coll Nutr. 2002;21(6):495–505.
20. Rubin MG, Kim K, Logan AC. Acne vulgaris, mental health and omega-3 fatty acids: a report of cases. Lipids Health Dis. 2008;7:36.
21. Koch C, Dölle S, Metzger M, Rasche C, Jungclas H, Rühl R, et al. Docosahexaenoic acid (DHA) supplementation in atopic eczema: a randomized, double-blind, controlled trial. Br J Dermatol. 2008;158(4):786–92.

22. Aslan İ, Özcan F, Karaarslan T, Kıraç E, Aslan M. Decreased eicosapentaenoic acid levels in acne vulgaris reveals the presence of a proinflammatory state. Prostaglandins Other Lipid Mediat. 2017;128–129:1–7.
23. Carta G, Murru E, Banni S, Manca C. Palmitic acid: physiological role, metabolism and nutritional implications. Front Physiol. 2017;8:902.
24. Annevelink CE, Sapp PA, Petersen KS, Shearer GC, Kris-Etherton PM. Diet-derived and diet-related endogenously produced palmitic acid: effects on metabolic regulation and cardiovascular disease risk. J Clin Lipidol. 2023;17(5):577–86.
25. Murru E, Manca C, Carta G, Banni S. Impact of dietary palmitic acid on lipid metabolism. Front Nutr. 2022;9:861664.
26. Grosso G, Galvano F, Marventano S, Malaguarnera M, Bucolo C, Drago F, et al. Omega-3 fatty acids and depression: scientific evidence and biological mechanisms. Oxidative Med Cell Longev. 2014;2014:313570.
27. Podgórska A, Puścion-Jakubik A, Markiewicz-Żukowska R, Gromkowska-Kępka KJ, Socha K. Acne vulgaris and intake of selected dietary nutrients—a summary of information. Healthcare (Basel). 2021;9(6):668.
28. Harwood JL. Polyunsaturated fatty acids: conversion to lipid mediators, roles in inflammatory diseases and dietary sources. Int J Mol Sci. 2023;24(10):8838.
29. Balić A, Vlašić D, Žužul K, Marinović B, Bukvić Mokos Z. Omega-3 versus omega-6 polyunsaturated fatty acids in the prevention and treatment of inflammatory skin diseases. Int J Mol Sci. 2020;21(3):741.
30. Guertler A, Neu K, Fiedler T, Kuna AC, Kämmerer T, Lill D, et al. Clinical effects of omega-3 fatty acids on acne vulgaris. J Dtsch Dermatol Ges. 2022;20(7):1023–7.
31. Serhan CN, Levy BD. Resolvins in inflammation: emergence of the pro-resolving superfamily of mediators. J Clin Invest. 2018;128(7):2657–69.
32. Ziboh VA. The significance of polyunsaturated fatty acids in cutaneous biology. Lipids. 1996;31(Suppl):S249–53.
33. Din JN, Newby DE, Flapan AD. Omega 3 fatty acids and cardiovascular disease—fishing for a natural treatment. BMJ. 2004;328(7430):30–5.
34. Williams-Bey Y, Boularan C, Vural A, Huang NN, Hwang IY, Shan-Shi C, et al. Omega-3 free fatty acids suppress macrophage inflammasome activation by inhibiting NF-κB activation and enhancing autophagy. PLoS One. 2014;9(6):e97957.
35. Macsai MS. The role of omega-3 dietary supplementation in blepharitis and meibomian gland dysfunction (an AOS thesis). Trans Am Ophthalmol Soc. 2008;106:336–56.
36. Surette ME, Koumenis IL, Edens MB, Tramposch KM, Chilton FH. Inhibition of leukotriene synthesis, pharmacokinetics, and tolerability of a novel dietary fatty acid formulation in healthy adult subjects. Clin Ther. 2003;25(3):948–71.
37. Jung JY, Kwon HH, Hong JS, Yoon JY, Park MS, Jang MY, et al. Effect of dietary supplementation with omega-3 fatty acid and gamma-linolenic acid on acne vulgaris: a randomised, double-blind, controlled trial. Acta Derm Venereol. 2014;94(5):521–5.
38. Hitch JM, Greenburg BG. Adolescent acne and dietary iodine. Arch Dermatol. 1961;84:898–911.
39. Cordain L, Lindeberg S, Hurtado M, Hill K, Eaton SB, Brand-Miller J. Acne vulgaris: a disease of Western civilization. Arch Dermatol. 2002;138(12):1584–90.
40. Simopoulos AP. The importance of the ratio of omega-6/omega-3 essential fatty acids. Biomed Pharmacother. 2002;56(8):365–79.

Microbiome Modulation: Probiotics, Prebiotics, and Postbiotics in Acne Vulgaris Therapy

5

Nereen A. Almosilhy and Esraa M. AlEdani

Contents

N. A. Almosilhy (✉)
Department of Pharmacology and Toxicology, Faculty of Pharmacy, Tanta University, Tanta, Egypt

E. M. AlEdani
Basra Medical College, Basrah, Iraq

E. M. AlEdani, H. I. Maibach (eds.), *Nutrition and Acne Vulgaris*, Updates in Clinical Dermatology, https://doi.org/10.1007/978-3-031-83677-0_5

5.1 Probiotics

Between 1845 and 1916, Ilya Ilyich Mechnikov, a winner of the Nobel Prize Russian zoologist, observed that long lifespans of Bulgarian peasants were associated with the consumption of lactic acid-producing bacteria in yogurt. This observation established the foundation for the incorporation of probiotics in the fields of health and medicine [1]. According to the World Health Organization (WHO) and the Food and Agriculture Organization (FAO), probiotics are defined as "live microorganisms that, when administered in adequate amounts, confer a health benefit on the host." [2]. Certain strains of anaerobic microbial genera such as *Lactobacillus*, *Bifidobacterium*, *Saccharomyces*, *Enterococcus*, *Streptococcus*, *Pediococcus*, *Leuconostoc*, and *Escherichia coli*, along with aerobic *Bacillus* strains, have been linked to beneficial aspects for human health [3].

5.1.1 Probiotics and Skin Health

Levkovich et al. [4] found that feeding mice yogurt containing *Lactobacillus reuteri* probiotics significantly improved their health, resulting in increased sebocytogenesis and folliculogenesis, which produced thicker, and shinier fur. The observed outcome was attributed to the probiotic's effects in regulating the immune system, particularly by enhancing the synthesis of the anti-inflammatory cytokine IL-10. As a result, regulatory T lymphocytes were produced and health-promoting hypothalamus hormones were secreted, which ultimately improved the integrity of the epithelial cells and increased immunological tolerance [4]. Nevertheless, the study did not investigate if the probiotic modified the gut microbiota composition, nor did it determine if comparable outcomes could be observed with other probiotics consumption. However, the results indicate possible advantages for the health of human skin, especially in cases of inflammatory skin conditions, given the prevalent co-existence of gut dysbiosis in these disorders. Probiotic strains that are widely available and have been the most extensively investigated are *Lactobacillus* and *Bifidobacteria*. They have shown beneficial impacts on skin health and can be found in various products, such as topical preparations, powders, supplements, and fermented dairy products [5].

5.1.2 Potential Molecular Mechanisms of Probiotics on the Skin

Potential therapeutic probiotics interventions in dermatology show promise through the interplay between the gastrointestinal tract and skin. Nevertheless, the exact molecular pathways responsible for this intercommunication remain poorly understood. The gut is acknowledged as a crucial immunological organ that contains the gut-associated lymphoid tissue (GALT), a complicated immune tissue that includes Peyer's patches [6]. These patches have a vital function in initiating immune responses in the mucosa. Dendritic cells located in Peyer's patches secrete IL-10 and influence the differentiation of T helper cells, which can result in the migration of these cytokines and activated immune cells to the skin, altering its immunological response and defense mechanisms [7]. Probiotics are believed to affect the immune system by interacting with Peyer's patches, potentially affecting skin health [8]. Moreover, the gut microbiota, with its extensive range of microorganisms, produces bioactive metabolites when it interacts with diet components. These metabolites are important signaling molecules that facilitate communication between the gut microbiota and the host [9]. Furthermore, UV light is a major factor in skin aging, leading to increased elasticity, dryness, and pigmentation by activating signaling pathways and transcribing target genes [10, 11]. Ultraviolet A (UVA) radiation enhances the generation of TNFα cytokine that promotes inflammation, in keratinocytes [12]. Research has investigated the potential of manipulating the gut microbiota to mitigate the damaging impacts of UV radiation. They found that Lipoteichoic acid (LTA), a *Lactobacillus* species' cell wall component, can reduce inflammation [12]. Furthermore, the administration of *Lactobacillus plantarum* HY7714 orally in mice and humans effectively reduced UV-induced photoaging, by suppressing the production of matrix metalloproteinase-1 (MMP-1), which is responsible for the degradation of collagen and other components of the extracellular matrix. Thus, enhancing skin elasticity and hydration [13, 14]. Also, different studies demonstrated that *Lactobacillus sakei* LTA was observed to modulate monocyte immune responses to counteract UV-induced skin aging [15].

5.2 Probiotics and Acne Vulgaris

Probiotics present a promising option for managing acne vulgaris by addressing the impact of intestinal dysbiosis on inflammatory skin conditions. They can be used as an alternative or supplementary therapy, avoiding the possible risks associated with antibiotic resistance and disruption of the microbiota, and potentially enhancing patient outcomes [16].

5.2.1 Pre-clinical Investigations on Probiotics Efficacy in Acne Vulgaris Treatment

Pre-clinical studies have demonstrated that different strains of probiotics can produce substances that hinder the growth of *C. acnes* and reduce inflammatory mediators, thereby potentially enhancing their efficacy in acne treatment (Table 5.1). Probiotics directly inhibit the growth of *C. acnes* with antimicrobial proteins. Specific strains, such as *Lactococcus* sp. HY449, *Streptococcus salivarius*, and *Enterococcus faecalis* release bacteriocins and bacteriocins-like inhibitory substances (BLIS) that impede the growth of *C. acnes*. In a study by Oh et al. [17] the antibacterial efficacy of bacteriocin generated by *Lactococcus* sp. HY 449 against various skin-inflammatory bacteria, such as *Staphylococcus aureus*, *Streptococcus pyogenes*, *Staphylococcus epidermidis*, and *Propionibacterium acnes*, was assessed.

Table 5.1 Pre-clinical studies on the effects of probiotics for acne treatment

Study name	Experimental design	Probiotic strain	Summary of study outcomes	Key findings
Oh et al. (2006) [17]	*In vitro*	*Lactococcus* sp. HY449	Assessed antibacterial efficacy of bacteriocin generated by *Lactococcus* sp. HY449 against skin-inflammatory bacteria.	Bacteriocin generated by Lactococcus sp. HY449 effectively suppressed *C. acnes*; no irritation or allergic responses in the human patch test.
Bowe et al. (2006) [18]	*In vitro*	*Streptococcus salivarius*	Swabs from 106 individuals were cultured to isolate *S. salivarius* and evaluate its BLIS production.	33.3% of isolates inhibited *C. acnes*; BLIS could be a natural antibiotic alternative.
Kang et al. (2009) [19]	*In vitro*	*Enterococcus faecalis* SL-5	Isolation of *Enterococcus faecalis SL-5* from human feces and testing its produced ESL5 bacteriocin antibacterial efficacy.	ESL5 bacteriocin significantly inhibited Gram-positive pathogens, including *C. acnes*.
Lee et al. (2012) [20]	*In vitro*	*Bifidobacterium adolescentis* SPM0308, *Bifidobacterium longum* SPM1207	Evaluated antibacterial and anti-inflammatory effects of 23 *Bifidobacterium* species.	Reduced survival of *C. acnes*; decreased macrophage production of inflammatory mediator.
Gueniche et al. (2010) [21]	*In vitro*	*Lactobacillus paracasei* CNCM I-2116 (ST11)	Investigated effects on skin inflammation.	Ameliorating substance P-induced mast cell degranulation and promoted skin barrier recovery.
Cosseau et al. (2008) [23]	*In vitro*	*Streptococcus salivarius K12*	Epithelial cells were cocultured with *Streptococcus salivarius* K12 or bacterial pathogens, to determine immune responses and cytokine secretion.	downregulated IL-8 secretion; promoted anti-inflammatory responses and maintained host-microbe balance.
Espinoza-Monje et al. (2021) [24]	*In vitro, In vivo*	*Weissella viridescens* UCO-SMC3	Investigated inhibition of *C. acnes* clinical isolates and immune response enhancement in mice through oral and topical *Weissella* formulations.	Significant inhibition of *C. acnes;* improved acne symptoms with topical application; oral administration modulated immune response.
Wang et al. (2014) [25]	*In vitro, In vivo*	*Staphylococcus epidermidis*	Studied glycerol fermentation and SCFAs production.	Succinic acid from fermentation inhibited *C. acnes* growth.

The findings demonstrated that the bacteriocin effectively suppressed the growth of all bacteria, with particularly rapid inactivated *C. acnes*. Bacteriocin's LC50 on human fibroblasts was 50 mg/mL, which did not affect the proliferation of normal cells. Moreover, no instances of irritation nor allergic responses were detected during a human patch test. This suggests that *Lactococcus* sp. HY 449 bacteriocin may be an effective antibiotic for suppressing *C. acnes* proliferation and preventing skin inflammation and acne when used as an antibacterial in cosmetic formulations.

Moreover, in a cross-sectional study by Bowe et al. [18], 106 individuals were recruited to provide swabs from the dorsum of the tongue, which were then cultured on mitis-salivarius agar to isolate *S. salivarius*. The *S. salivarius* isolates were examined for their ability to suppress the growth of *C. acnes* and Group A *Streptococcus* (GAS) through the generation of BLIS. They found that *C. acnes* was inhibited by 11 isolates (33.3%), while GAS was inhibited by 13 isolates (39.4%), and five strains generated bacteriocins that had inhibitory effects on both *C. acnes* and GAS. The findings suggest that the BLIS produced by *S. salivarius* may serve as a natural substitute for antibiotics in the treatment of acne, potentially mitigating the development of antibiotic resistance. Another study by Kang et al. [19] isolated *Enterococcus faecalis* SL-5 from human feces. This lactic acid bacterial strain significantly inhibited Gram-positive pathogens, including *C. acnes*, by producing an antibacterial agent identified as a bacteriocin known as ESL5.

Interestingly, an *in vitro* study investigated the antibacterial and anti-inflammatory effects of 23 *Bifidobacterium* species as potential probiotics. The researchers observed that certain *Bifidobacterium* strains exhibited antibacterial activity against *Staphylococcus aureus* and *Propionibacterium acnes*. Specifically, six sonicated *Bifidobacterium* strains were found to inhibit *Staphylococcus aureus*. In contrast, the survival of *C. acnes* was dramatically reduced by two strains: *Bifidobacterium adolescentis* SPM0308 and *Bifidobacterium longum* SPM1207. Furthermore, the study assessed the anti-inflammatory effects of these two strains, either in live form or as cell-free supernatants. The results revealed a significant decrease in macrophage production of inflammatory mediators, including nitric oxide and TNF-α, compared to the control group. Another *in vitro* study by Gueniche et al. [21] concluded that *Lactobacillus paracasei* CNCM I-2116 (ST11) effectively controls skin inflammation by ameliorating substance P-induced mast cell degranulation, vasodilation, edema, and TNF-alpha production. Additionally, it promoted the recovery of skin barrier function, in an *ex-vivo* skin culture, recommending its usage as an oral supplement to treat inflammatory skin diseases, including acne vulgaris.

In addition, probiotics can modify the immune response of keratinocytes and epithelial cells. For example, *in vitro* studies showed that cocultured human epithelial cells with *S. salivarius* strain K12; prevented the production of pro-inflammatory cytokines such as IL-8, did not induce proinflammatory responses, stimulated anti-inflammatory responses, and modulated genes associated with adhesion and homeostasis [23]. Moreover, the probiotic strain NCC2461 (ST11/CNCM I-2116) has been shown to help restore homeostasis by modulating both mucosal and systemic immunity. While the gut-skin connection remains unclear, studies show that NCC2461 benefits skin health by strengthening the skin barrier, reducing sensitivity, and regulating immune responses, ultimately contributing to skin homeostasis [22]. Espinoza-Monje et al. [24] found that *Weissella viridescens* UCO-SMC3 inhibited *C. acnes* clinical isolates and reduced its keratinocyte adhesion in *in vitro* studies. Additionally, their *in vivo* experiments demonstrated that both oral and topical *Weissella viridescens* UCO-SMC3 treatment boosted the immune response and reduced *C. acnes* growth in lesions. As in the oral administration resulted in a higher modulation of the immune response against *C. acnes* compared to topical therapy. Conversely, topical administration was more effective than oral treatment in reducing bacterial loads on the skin, likely due to its ability to hinder *C. acnes* adherence [24].

Another intriguing study by Wang et al. [25] found that glycerol fermentation by the human skin microbiome, specifically by *Staphylococcus epidermidis*, produces short chain fatty acids (SCFAs) such as succinic acid which effectively creates an inhospitable environment for the overgrowth of *C. acnes* both *in vitro* and *in vivo*. The findings demonstrate the potential of employing fermentation in developing probiotics for treating acne and highlight the effectiveness of succinic acid as a therapeutic agent to combat *C. acnes* inflammation and proliferation [25].

5.3 Clinical Evidence on Probiotic Efficacy in Acne Vulgaris Treatment

5.3.1 Oral Probiotics for Acne Vulgaris Treatment

Research on the effectiveness of probiotics as a treatment for acne vulgaris in humans is relatively limited; however, several clinical trials have shown promising results for probiotics in acne therapy (Table 5.2). In 1961, Union Memorial Hospital physician Robert H. Sawyer published the first official clinical report on probiotics' potential benefits by following 300 patients who received commercial probiotic tablets, Lactinex®, containing a combination of *L. acidophilus* and *L. bulgaricus*, he detected a significant clinical improvement in 80% of acne patients, especially in inflammatory acne cases. Furthermore, Sawyer observed correlations between acne skin manifestations and the metabolic processes of the gastrointestinal tract. However, the study lacked a control or placebo group for comparison. In 1987, an Italian trial involved 20 patients who consumed 250 mg oral probiotic supplement containing freeze-dried *L. acidophilus* and *Bifidobacterium bifidum* as adjuvant therapy had better lesion repair, clinical responses, and oral antibiotic tolerance than 20 patients not receiving the supplements. Likewise, in a Russian study, patients who received intestinal microflora-correcting agents alongside conventional acne treatments exhibited faster clinical improvements. Additionally, over a 12-week trial, Kim et al. [29] observed that the consumption of a fermented dairy *Lactobacillus* probiotic drink by acne patients significantly reduced inflammatory and total lesions, acne severity, sebum content, triacylglycerols, and free fatty acids on the skin. While the supplementation of lactoferrin, an anti-inflammatory and bactericidal milk

Table 5.2 Clinical trials on the treatment of acne vulgaris with oral probiotics

Study name	Study design	Probiotic strain	Summary of study outcomes	Key findings
Siver (1961) [26]	Observational clinical trial	*L. acidophilus, L. bulgaricus*	Followed 300 patients using Lactinex® probiotic tablets.	Significant clinical improvement in 80% of acne patients and correlations between acne skin manifestations and the GI metabolic processes.
Marchetti et al. (1987) [27]	Observational clinical trial	*L. acidophilus, Bifidobacterium bifidum*	Compared probiotic supplements to control in acne treatment.	Better lesion repair and clinical responses with probiotic supplements compared to control.
Volkova et al. (2001) [28]	Observational clinical trial	Various strains	Examined effects of intestinal microflora-correcting agents on acne.	Faster clinical improvements were observed.
Kim et al. (2010) [29]	Observational clinical trial	*Lactobacillus* strains	Evaluated lactoferrin-enriched fermented dairy drink effects on skin surface lipids and symptoms of acne vulgaris.	Reduced inflammatory and total lesions; decreased sebum content, triacylglycerols, and free fatty acids on the skin.
Rahmayani et al. (2019) [31]	pretest-posttest clinical trial	Various strains	Measured serum IL-10 levels in 33 acne patients who consumed oral probiotics for a month.	Significant increase in IL-10 levels, suggesting reduced inflammation.
Jung et al. (2013) [33]	RCT	*Lactobacillus* strains	Assessed minocycline regimen for treating acne with and without probiotics.	The greatest reduction in lesion count was with probiotics and minocycline combination.
Fabbrocini et al. (2016) [32]	Pilot RCT	*Lactobacillus rhamnosus* GG (LGG)	Examined effects of IGF-1 regulation in 20 acne adult patients.	Clinical improvement in acne by modulating gut-skin axis and insulin signaling.

(continued)

Table 5.2 (continued)

Study name	Study design	Probiotic strain	Summary of study outcomes	Key findings
Manzhalii et al. (2016) [30]	RCT	*Escherichia coli Nissle 1917 (EcN)*	Investigated effects of Mutaflor® tablets on 82 patients with facial dermatoses.	Normalized IgA levels, reduced IL-8, preserved the mucosal barrier through favorable gut microbiota overgrowth, and improved patient quality of life.
Tolino et al. (2018) [34]	RCT	Various strains	Evaluated a complete skincare line with topical cream device and/or gender-specific oral supplements.	Significant improvements in acne grading scores; most improvement in the oral supplement groups.
Rinaldi et al. (2022) [35]	RCT	*Ligilactobacillus salivarius* LS03, *Lactaseibacillus casei* LC03, *Bifidobacterium breve* BR03	Investigated dysbiosis-associated acne by comparing probiotic mixture, botanical extract, and their combinations.	Probiotic-botanical extract supplement was most effective in reducing acne symptoms and microbial dysbiosis.
Eguren et al. (2024) [36]	RCT	*Arthrospira platensis* (BEA_IDA_0074B), *Lacticaseibacillus rhamnosus* (CECT 30031)	Evaluated the efficacy of oral probiotics in 74 patients with acne vulgaris.	Improved clinical outcomes and non-inflammatory lesions.

protein, further decreased inflammatory lesions, the distinct benefits of the probiotic drink alone suggest that probiotics may be an effective adjunct treatment for acne.

The probiotic bacteria inhibit the activity of the proinflammatory cytokine as interleukin-8 in epithelial cells and keratinocytes, leading to an immunoregulatory effect. Moreover, these microorganisms do not cause proinflammatory reactions; instead, they stimulate anti-inflammatory effects and regulate genes associated with epithelial adhesion molecules and homeostasis. Also, they suppress other bacteria without affecting the skin microbiome, providing antibiotic-like benefits without adverse effects. Thus, probiotics, as immunoregulators, have demonstrated notable effectiveness in treating Grade III and IV acne, which are associated with severe inflammation. The effects of oral administration of *Escherichia coli Nissle* 1917 (EcN) (Mutaflor®) were investigated in an RCT comprising 82 patients suffering from facial dermatoses such as acne, seborrhoeic dermatitis, and papular-pustular rosacea. The researchers reported that EcN therapy normalized IgA levels, reduced the pro-inflammatory cytokine IL-8, and improved quality of life. Additionally, the experimental group showed a positive shift in microbiota composition, with increased levels of beneficial *bifidobacteria* and *lactobacteria* and decreased pathogenic bacteria. Therefore, the study emphasizes the potential of EcN therapy as a new and innovative treatment method by preserving the mucosal barrier through favorable gut microbiota overgrowth, modulating the immune response, and improving clinical outcomes in patients with intestinal-borne dermatoses. Moreover, in a pre-experimental clinical investigation with a pretest-posttest design involving 33 patients with acne vulgaris, oral probiotics were consumed for 30 days, and serum IL-10 levels were evaluated before and after the intervention. The study results showed a significant increase in IL-10 levels post-administration, suggesting that probiotics might mitigate inflammation through the generation of regulatory cytokines such as IL-10.

Fabbrocini et al. [32] performed an interesting pilot RCT that found that probiotics modulate insulin-like growth factor 1 (IGF-1), which contributes to acne pathogenesis. They concluded that a daily dose of the probiotic strain *Lactobacillus rhamnosus* GG (LGG) clinically improved the appearance of acne in 20 participants over 12 weeks. This improvement was achieved by normalizing the skin gene expression of the insulin signaling-related IGF1 and FOXO1 genes. The findings suggest that probiotics may modulate the gut-skin axis, thereby affecting systemic inflammation and insulin signaling. Additionally, Jung et al. [33] conducted a prospective open-label RCT to evaluate the safety, efficacy, and tolerability of a minocycline regimen for treating acne, with and without probiotics supplementation. They found a synergistic anti-inflammatory effect when combining probiotics with minocycline, while also mitigating the potential risks associated with long-term antibiotic use.

Furthermore, in a double-blinded clinical trial with equal numbers of men and women, the efficacy and tolerability of a complete skincare line for mild to moderate acne were evaluated using the Global Acne Grading System (GAGS). The regimen included a topical cream device comprising active plant agents, keratolytic molecules and distinct gender-specific oral supplements containing biotin, probiotics, vitamin E, zinc, and nicotinamide, with beta-sitosterol and Boswellia serrata added for men, and myo-inositol and folic acid for women. All groups demonstrated significant improvements in GAGS scores, with the oral supplement groups showing the most substantial improvement, suggesting a novel and effective treatment for mild to moderate acne. Rinaldi et al. [35] conducted an 8-week, four-arm, placebo-controlled, double-blind RCT involving 114 patients with mild to moderate acne to investigate dysbiosis associated acne and examine alternatives to topical and systemic antibiotics. The trial results showed that the probiotic mixture (*Ligilactobacillus salivarius* LS03, *Lactobacillus casei* LC03, and *Bifidobacterium breve* BR03), botanical extracts (Lupeol and Echinacea), or their combination significantly reduced facial acne lesion count (GAGS score), desquamation rate, sebum production, erythema, porphyrins, and microbial dysbiosis compared to placebo. The probiotic-botanical extract supplement had the most beneficial effects, suggesting it may be a safe and effective adjuvant therapy for inflammatory acne and acne-prone skin. Recently, in 2024, a 12-week RCT involving 74 patients with mild-to-moderate acne evaluated the efficacy of an oral probiotic containing

Arthrospira platensis (BEA_IDA_0074B) and *Lacticaseibacillus rhamnosus* (CECT 30031) compared to a placebo. Investigators found that 50% of patients in the probiotic group improved on the Acne Global Severity Scale (AGSS), compared to 29.41% of those in the placebo group. Additionally, the oral probiotic formula ameliorated non-inflammatory lesions and increased the GAGS score by 42.50%, compared to 20.58% in the placebo group.

5.3.2 Topical Probiotics for Acne Vulgaris Treatment

In 1912, Peyri conducted a pioneering study on the potential benefits of applying *L. bulgaricus* locally to treat acne and seborrhoea, which laid the foundation for the concept of 'topical bacteriotherapy' [37]. However, it was not until 1999 that Di Marzio et al. expanded on this concept by demonstrating that applying a cream containing *Streptococcus thermophilus*, a species commonly found in yogurt, to the skin for a week could significantly increase ceramide synthesis [38]. Ceramides strengthen the skin's barrier, allowing for better water retention and relief from irritation caused by topical agents [39]. This important finding has been confirmed in several subsequent studies [40, 41]. Ceramide sphingolipids particularly phyto-sphingosine (PS) possess direct anti-inflammatory effects and antibacterial properties against *C. acnes* [42]. Thus, a 2-month pilot trial found that 0.2% PS topical application decreased pustules and papules by 89%. Moreover, clinical trials have reported that *Lactobacillus plantarum* significantly reduced mild acne lesions and erythema and improved skin barrier repair. The probiotic extract was sterilized and filtered before being included in an aqueous lotion at concentrations of 1% and 5%. Then, a group of ten individuals, ranging in age from 18 to 50 years, applied the lotion once daily for 4 days. The application of the 5% concentration resulted in a significant reduction in both lesion size and erythema, while the 1% concentration did not exhibit any significant effects. The study recommended the 5% formulation for treating mild acne, demonstrating the dose-dependent efficacy of *lactobacilli* [43]. Furthermore, Espinoza-Monje et al. [24] conducted a clinical pilot study that demonstrated significant improvements in acne symptoms after applying a face cream containing *W. viridescens* UCO-SMC3 nightly for 5 weeks [24]. Also, Sathikulpakdee et al. [44] conducted an RCT with 104 patients to assess the efficacy and safety of a lotion containing *Lactobacillus paracasei* MSMC 39-1 and 2.5% benzoyl peroxide for the treatment of mild to moderate acne vulgaris. The study found that the probiotic lotion was as effective as benzoyl peroxide in treating inflammatory acne lesions and reducing erythema, with fewer adverse effects, making it a suitable alternative for patients allergic to benzoyl peroxide(Table 5.3) [44].

Table 5.3 Clinical trials on the treatment of acne vulgaris with topical probiotics

Study name	Study design	Probiotic strain	Summary of study outcomes	Key findings
Peyri (1912) [37]	Case study	*L. bulgaricus*	Early study on topical application for acne and seborrhoea.	Laid foundation for topical bacteriotherapy.
Di Marzio et al. (1999, 2003, 2008) [38, 40, 41]	Observational trial	*Streptococcus thermophilus*	Applied cream containing *S. thermophilus*; assessed ceramide synthesis.	Increased ceramide synthesis, strengthening the skin barrier.
Muizzuddin et al. (2012) [43]	Observational trial	*Lactobacillus plantarum*	Applied lotion containing *L. plantarum* to acne patients.	Significant reduction in lesion size and erythema.
Espinoza-Monje et al. (2021) [24]	Pilot Observational trial	*Weissella viridescens* UCO-SMC3	Applying a face cream containing *W. viridescens* UCO-SMC3 nightly for 5 weeks to acne patients.	Significant improvements in acne symptoms.
Sathikulpakdee et al. (2022) [44]	RCT	*Lactobacillus paracasei* MSMC 39–1	Compared probiotic lotion to benzoyl peroxide treatment for acne.	Probiotic lotion was as effective as benzoyl peroxide with fewer adverse reactions.

5.4 Prebiotics

Gibson and Roberfroid first proposed the concept of prebiotics in 1995 through their investigation of the impact of dietary modulation on the human intestinal microbiota. They defined a prebiotic as a non-digestible food ingredient that benefits the host's health by selectively promoting the growth and/or activity of certain gut bacteria. This definition remained unchanged for 15 years, and according to it, only a few carbohydrate molecules, including lactulose, inulin, fructo-oligosaccharide (FOS), and galacto-oligosaccharides (GOS), were categorized as prebiotics [45]. However, the International Scientific Association for Probiotics and Prebiotics (ISAPP) recently redefined dietary prebiotics as substrates that are specifically utilized by host microorganisms to provide a health benefit. This updated definition encompasses non-carbohydrate compounds and extends its applications beyond the gastrointestinal system. Moreover, this definition is also applicable to animal prebiotics [46]. Prebiotics are naturally found in various sources such as asparagus, sugar beet, honey, garlic, onion, chicory, Jerusalem artichoke, tomato, wheat, banana, barley, soybean, beans, peas, human and cow's milk, rye, and recently, microalgae and seaweeds. However, due to their low concentrations in natural sources, prebiotics are often mass-produced industrially using lactose, sucrose, and starch [47–49].

5.4.1 Types of Prebiotics

There are several different types of prebiotics, which primarily consist of carbohydrates, specifically oligosaccharide carbohydrates (OSCs). These include:

I. Fructans, such as inulin and fructo-oligosaccharide (FOS) (often called oligofructose), are known to activate lactic acid bacteria [50]. Research indicates that the length of the fructan chain affects which bacteria can ferment them, suggesting a potential to promote various bacteria either directly or indirectly [51].

II. Galacto-oligosaccharides (GOS) are divided into two categories: those with excess galactose at specific sites and those produced by enzymatic trans-glycosylation of lactose, known as trans-galacto-oligosaccharides (TOS) [52, 53]. GOS stimulates the growth of *Bifidobacteria* and *Lactobacilli*, particularly *Bifidobacteria* in infants while exerting a lesser influence on other microbial taxa such as *Enterobacteria*, *Bacteroidetes*, and *Firmicutes* [50]. Certain types of GOS originate from lactulose, which is the isomer of lactose and is also recognized as prebiotics [53]. Another form of GOS, raffinose family oligosaccharides (RFO), is based on sucrose extension, however, its impact on gut microbiota remains unclear [54, 55].

III. Glucose-derived oligosaccharides and resistant starch (RS), researchers determined that RS which resists upper digestive system processing, may serve as a prebiotic by increasing the levels of butyrate, which is beneficial for health [56]. An *in vitro* study by Ze et al. [57] investigated the impact of four prevalent amylolytic bacteria in the human colon on the processing of RS and showed that *Bacteroides thetaiotaomicron* and *Eubacterium rectale* had limited ability compared to *Bifidobacterium adolescentis* and *Ruminococcus bromii*. They also discovered that the breakdown of RS in mixed bacterial and fecal incubations requires the presence of *R. bromii* [57]. Furthermore, several types of *Firmicutes* have shown the greatest levels of incorporation when exposed to abundant RS [58]. Additionally, in a human-feeding, placebo-controlled, double-blind crossover trial exploring the effects of Polydextrose (PDX), glucose-derived oligosaccharides, on the composition of colonic microbiota, investigators found that PDX significantly enhances butyrate-producing *Ruminococcus intestinalis* and bacteria from *Clostridium clusters* I, II, and IV while reducing levels of *Lactobacillus–Enterococcus* [59].

IV. Other oligosaccharides in plant cell walls, derived from polysaccharides such as pectin, are referred to as pectic oligosaccharides (POS) and are considered promising sources for prebiotic production [60, 61].

V. Non-carbohydrate oligosaccharides: Although most of the relevant literature primarily focuses on oligosaccharides (OSCs), there is also data indicating that prebiotics encompass a broader range beyond carbohydrates. Non-carbohydrate oligosaccharides, such as cocoa-derived flavanols, have been shown in both *in vivo* and *in vitro* studies to activate lactic acid bacteria [62].

5.4.2 Prebiotics and Human Health

However, the available literature on prebiotics' effects on human health is scarce compared to that on probiotics, and several studies often combined prebiotics with probiotics. Nevertheless, prebiotics have demonstrated their ability to enhance health via multiple mechanisms [63]. Intestinal bacteria break down (ferment) prebiotics, resulting in alterations to the composition and activity of gut bacteria, favoring beneficial bacteria (e.g. *bifidobacteria* and *lactobacilli*), promoting gut barrier function, improving SCFA synthesis, modulating the immune system, and suppressing pathogenic bacteria (e.g. *Listeria monocytogens*, *E. coli*, *Salmonella typhimurium*, *Clostridium perfringens*, *S. aureus*, and *C. acnes*) [64–73].

Furthermore, prebiotics might prevent colorectal cancer by promoting the growth of SCFAs-producing bacteria, rather than those that produce carcinogenic compounds [74]. Prebiotic effects on the gut can also extend to affect other organs such as the skin, vagina, and bladder [70, 75–77]. Moreover, various studies have reported the efficacy of prebiotics such as GOS, FOS, inulin, and Konjac glucomannan in reducing inflammation and alleviating symptoms associated with inflammatory bowel disease (IBD), atopic dermatitis (AD), allergic rhinitis, and other inflammatory conditions [69, 78–82]. Prebiotics enhance mineral bioavailability, particularly calcium and magnesium, and positively influence lipid and hepatic metabolism by reducing blood lipids such as triacylglycerol (TAG) and very low-density lipoprotein (VLDL) while increasing high-density lipoprotein (HDL) levels [83, 84]. They also affect the levels of hormones like ghrelin and peptide YY, which regulate hunger and food intake, thereby promoting satiety, weight management, and preventing obesity [85].

5.4.3 Prebiotics and Skin Health

Researchers have found that GOS increases the expression of CD44 and collagen type 1, markers of cell adhesion, and matrix formation, thereby improving the skin barrier. Additionally, the metabolism of aromatic amino acids by intestinal microorganisms produces phenols, such as p-cresol, which are harmful to kidney patients and can be transferred to the skin. However, investigations showed that GOS—either alone or combined with probiotics—may prevent phenol-induced water and keratin loss [86–88]. Hong et al. [89] discovered that hairless mice treated with GOS and *Bifidobacterium longum* for 12 weeks retained more water and were protected against UV-induced erythema [89]. Additionally, Akiyama et al. [90] found that GOS can effectively reduce *S. aureus* proliferation, which often infects or colonizes the horny cells of AD lesions, thereby preventing the exacerbation of these lesions [90].

Moreover, prebiotics can reduce the severity and risk of allergic skin disorders, including AD, in infants, as demonstrated in two RCTs. Grüber et al. [91] employed a formula containing neutral and pectin-derived acidic oligosaccharides, while Moro et al. [78] utilized a mixture of galacto- and long-chain fructo-oligosaccharides [78, 91]. Another RCT investigated the effects of orally administered Triphala, a polyphenol-rich prebiotic, on 80 participants with scalp seborrhea. The trial showed that Triphala significantly reduced scalp sebum levels compared to a placebo. Additionally, Triphala was well-tolerated and increased patient satisfaction, highlighting its potential in managing scalp seborrhea [92].

Prebiotics exhibit low dosage efficacy, lack adverse effects, and demonstrate intestinal persistence [93]. However, prebiotics vary in solubility in different skincare formulations, presenting several challenges [76]. Moreover, maintaining the prebiotics or probiotics functions and effectiveness through skin contact is challenging due to factors such as hygiene, clothing, and environmental exposure. Nonetheless, in contrast to probiotics, prebiotics retain their efficacy in formulations because of the relative stability of their carbohydrate components, unlike other topical components [94].

5.4.4 Prebiotics in Acne Vulgaris Treatment

Despite the limited literature on the effects of prebiotics on acne vulgaris, prebiotics have shown a significant role in acne management in various studies [70, 95, 96]. Dall'Oglio et al. [96] conducted a pilot study involving 12 women with mild to moderate acne, which revealed that oral supplementation with FOS and GOS prebiotics improves glycemic and lipid metabolism. This indicates that prebiotics could potentially manage acne through metabolic modulation [96]. Another recent multicenter RCT revealed that oral prebiotic food supplements containing FOS&GOS, zinc, niacinamide, and lactoferrin, along with a topical cream containing retinoid molecules, Iris Florentina root extract, and oligopeptides, are effective and well-tolerated in 184 women with acne. The combination significantly decreased the inflammatory lesions and reduced scores on both the Global Acne Severity Scale (GEA) and the Adult Female Acne Scoring Tool (AFAST) [95]. Konjac glucomannan hydrolysates (GMH), a polysaccharide extracted from the tubers of Asian *Amorphophallus* species, combined with probiotics in an *in vitro* study have been also shown to enhance the inhibition of *C. acnes* growth compared to probiotics alone, suggesting their potential in acne management [70].

5.5 Synbiotics

A synbiotic combines probiotics and prebiotics to synergically improve health by increasing probiotic strain viability and colonization [93, 97]. In an *in vivo* study by Su et al. [98], mice treated with inulin, FOS, and soybean oligosaccharide (SOS) demonstrated increased survival and retention of *lactobacillus acidophilus* LAFTI®

L10, *lactobacillus casei* L26 LAFTI, and *Bifidobacterium lactis* LAFTI® B94, suggesting potential use in developing synbiotic pharmaceutical and food products [98]. Probiotic strains frequently included in synbiotic preparations are derived from the *Lactobacillus*, *Streptococcus*, *Bifidobacterium*, and *Enterococcus* genera. These formulations contain various important prebiotics, including FOS, GOS, inulin, transgalactooligosaccharides, xylooligosaccharides, lactitol, lactulose, and lactosucrose [93, 99, 100].

Numerous studies have examined the health impacts of synbiotics, particularly in the metabolic improvements of type 2 diabetic (DM) patients, weight management in obese individuals, gut microbiome modulation, treatment and prevention of gastrointestinal disorders such as irritable bowel syndrome (IBS), and various skin conditions including acne vulgaris [82, 101–110]. Synbiotics optimize, maintain, and restore skin microbiota systemically or topically. A significant challenge with topical probiotic applications, even in synbiotic formulations, is the harsh skin environment, which limits colonization [111]. Nonetheless, other parts of the body, such as the mouth and vagina, where beneficial microbial populations are present, are not affected by this issue [76, 112].

5.6 Postbiotics

Several studies suggested that dead probiotic cells can produce beneficial biological responses when administered orally or topically in sufficient amounts, similar to their live equivalents [113, 114]. As they cannot be classified as probiotics, new terms such as postbiotics, paraprobiotics, inactivated probiotics, non-viable probiotics, ghost probiotics, and tyndallized probiotics have been introduced [115–117]. According to the ISAPP, postbiotics are defined as "a preparation of inanimate microorganisms and/or their components that benefit the host." [118]. Therefore, postbiotics are microbes' fragments or metabolites that directly or indirectly benefit the host without containing live bacteria; hence, they cannot multiply. This includes cell wall fragments, cell-free supernatants, exopolysaccharides (EPSs), bacterial lysates (BLs), enzymes, SCFAs, vitamins, and phenolic compounds [119, 120]. The heterogeneity of postbiotic structures suggests that the inactivation techniques of viable cells can be achieved through various mechanical and chemical methods, including sonication, thermal treatment, high pressure, electromagnetic radiation, ultraviolet irradiation, solvent extraction, enzymatic extraction, chromatography, and dialysis. Notably, purified metabolites and cell components have distinct chemical identities and are not considered postbiotics but rather microbe-derived compounds [121, 122]. Postbiotics, which do not contain live microbes, promote health through mechanisms similar to probiotics while reducing associated risks. Like prebiotics, postbiotics have minimal adverse effects and are effective as probiotics, although no research has yet compared the two groups directly [122]. Currently, the available literature does not classify postbiotics as synbiotics; as previously shown, synbiotics are a combination of prebiotics and probiotics that modulate the gut microbiome [123]. Postbiotics have been shown in various studies to improve the intestinal microbiome, suggesting that the definition of "synbiotics" should expanded to include them [122].

5.6.1 Postbiotics: Beyond Probiotics and Prebiotics

A defined chemical composition, the inability to transfer antibiotic-resistance genes or virulence factors, and the lack of exposure to live microorganisms make postbiotics much safer than probiotics, especially for immunosuppressed patients and children with immature immune systems and disturbed intestinal barriers [124, 125]. Furthermore, postbiotics have a longer shelf life and lack concerns of bacteremia and fungemia, while maintaining stability in industrial operations and under external conditions such as UV light, oxidation, varying temperatures, and pH levels [118]. As with probiotics and prebiotics, postbiotics are usually encapsulated for oral consumption or formulated as topical creams [126, 127]. Although probiotics have unpredictable production and dose standardization concerns, postbiotics do not. In fact, they allow for repetitive production processes and precise quantitative control [122]. Since they do not require viable cells in the formula, postbiotics are more cost-effective to store and transport [128].

5.6.2 Postbiotics and Skin Health

Even though the field of postbiotics is relatively new and research on their applications and efficacy remains limited, recent investigations have demonstrated their significant effectiveness in skin moisturization and wrinkle prevention, as well as in treating various skin conditions, including atopic dermatitis, acne vulgaris, alopecia, and wound healing [129–138].

5.6.3 Postbiotics in Acne Vulgaris Treatment

Several recent studies have shown the safety and efficacy of postbiotics as adjuvant therapy in the treatment of acne vulgaris (Table 5.4) [136, 137, 139–142]. Majeed et al. [137, 138] investigated the dermal-protective effects of LactoSporin®, a purified extracellular metabolite from the fermented broth of *Bacillus coagulans* MTCC 5856, in *in vitro* studies. They revealed its antioxidant, anti-inflammatory, anti-aging properties, and antimicrobial activity against *C. acnes, S. epidermidis,* and *S. aureus*, as well as its ability to inhibit the 5-alpha reductase enzyme, which is involved in sebum production 137, 138. Furthermore, Majeed and his colleagues supported the *in vitro* findings with a 3-week RCT involving 64 patients with mild-to-moderate acne to compare the safety and efficacy of LactoSporin® 2% cream with benzoyl peroxide 2.5% gel. The results showed that the efficacy of LactoSporin® 2% cream was comparable to that of benzoyl peroxide 2.5% gel in treating mild-to-moderate acne. However, LactoSporin® had a faster onset of action in reducing closed

Table 5.4 Studies on the treatment of acne vulgaris with postbiotics

Study name	Study design	Used postbiotic	Summary of study outcomes	Key findings
Majeed et al. (2020) [137, 138]	*In vitro*, RCT	LactoSporin®	Investigated antioxidant, anti-inflammatory, anti-aging, and antimicrobial properties; safety and efficacy on RCT compared to benzoyl peroxide	LactoSporin® 2% cream comparable to benzoyl peroxide 2.5% gel; faster onset of action in reducing closed comedones; more effective in reducing sebum and oiliness; non-irritant
Cui et al. (2022) [141]	Observational pilot study	*Lactiplantibacillus plantarum* VHProbi E15 ferment lysate	Evaluated the safety and efficacy of anti-acne lotion containing *Lactiplantibacillus plantarum* VHProbi E15 lysate	Increased skin hydration, reduced acne lesions, controlled sebum production
Cui et al. (2022) [142]	Observational study	*Lactiplantibacillus plantarum* VHProbi V22 ferment lysate	Evaluated safety and efficacy of anti-acne cream containing *Lactiplantibacillus plantarum* VHProbi V22 lysate	Similar results to the VHProbi E15 lysate study
Kang et al. (2022) [143]	RCT	*Enterococcus faecalis* CBT SL-5	Evaluated lotion containing CBT SL-5 on patients with acne	Reduced pustules compared to placebo lotion
Han et al. (2022) [144]	Split-face RCT	*Enterococcus faecalis* CBT SL-5	Evaluated lotion containing CBT SL-5 on patients with acne compared to placebo lotion	Reduced acne severity and skin microbiome dysbiosis; equivalent transepidermal water loss and skin hydration between groups
Chung et al. (2022) [136]	*In vitro*	Postbiotic Complex (PC) from cell-free supernatants of *Lactococcus lactis* (HY449) and *Lactobacillus helveticus* (HY7801)	Evaluated antibacterial and anti-inflammatory properties against *C. acnes* and *S. aureus* on human keratinocytes	Demonstrated antibacterial and anti-inflammatory properties; attributed to specific metabolites identified through GC-MS

(continued)

Table 5.4 (continued)

Study name	Study design	Used postbiotic	Summary of study outcomes	Key findings
Ho et al. (2022) [140]	Observational study	Collagen co-fermented with (TYCA06/AP-32/CP-9, TAC)	Evaluated antimicrobial and anti-inflammatory effects of a TAC/Collagen gel on acne patient	Inhibited *C. acnes* growth, reduced inflammation, improved wound healing, enhanced acne symptoms, and skin condition
Bae et al. (2023) [139]	Single-arm clinical trial	Heat-treated *Pediococcus acidilactici* LM1013 (HT-LM1013)	Investigated efficacy of HT-LM1013 as a daily leave-on product for treating acne vulgaris	Inhibited *C. acnes* biofilm development, reduced lipase activity, decreased comedone count and sebum production, with high patient satisfaction

comedones, visible as early as 3 days, and was more effective in reducing sebum secretion and oiliness. Both treatments were safe and well-tolerated, with LactoSporin® being notably non-irritant [138]. This suggests its promising role in treating acne and potentially other seborrheic conditions [137, 138].

Cui et al. [141] performed a 1-month pilot study on the safety and efficacy of an anti-acne lotion containing *Lactiplantibacillus plantarum* VHProbi E15 ferment lysate. The results demonstrated that the anti-acne lotion increased skin hydration, reduced acne lesions, and controlled sebum production [141]. In a separate observational study, Cui and another group [142] evaluated the safety and efficacy of an anti-acne cream containing *Lactiplantibacillus plantarum* VHProbi V22 lysate, which reported similar results [142]. Moreover, Kang et al. [143] formed a lotion containing a concentrated powder of the cell-free culture supernatant (CFCS) of *E. faecalis* SL-5 (CBT SL-5) that was evaluated on patients with mild to moderate acne. CBT SL-5 lotion showed reduced pustules compared to placebo lotion, displaying that *E. faecalis* SL-5 may be an option with topical antibiotics for acne treatment [143]. Another investigation examined the effects of a lotion containing *E. faecalis* CBT SL-5 extract in a 20-person, randomized, placebo-controlled, split-face trial over 4 weeks. Participants applied *E. faecalis* lotion on one side of their face and a placebo carrier lotion on the other. Compared to the placebo, the *E. faecalis* lotion dramatically reduced acne severity and skin microbiome dysbiosis in mild-to-moderate acne patients. Nonetheless, both groups experienced equivalent transepidermal water loss and skin hydration [144].

Chung et al. [136] developed a Postbiotic Complex (PC) utilizing cell-free supernatants derived from *Lactococcus lactis* (HY449) and *Lactobacillus helveticus* (HY7801) probiotic strains. Their approach included multiple strains due to the limitation of a single strain in achieving all desired biological effects. Upon assessment against *C. acnes* and *S. aureus*, both of which are known to be involved in common skin conditions like acne and atopic dermatitis, the PC demonstrated antibacterial and anti-inflammatory properties on human keratinocytes. The observed effect was attributed to specific metabolites, rather than acidic properties. These metabolites, including hypoxanthine, ornithine, 2-hydroxyisocaproic acid, succinic acid, and γ-aminobutyric acid (GABA), were identified through the analysis of postbiotic metabolic profiles using GC-MS [136]. Another interesting clinical study by Ho et al. [140] evaluated the antimicrobial and anti-inflammatory effects of a cosmetic gel containing collagen co-fermented with three probiotic strains (TYCA06/AP-32/CP-9, TAC) for treating acne vulgaris. Participants applied the gel on different sides of their faces twice daily. The co-fermented TAC/Collagen postbiotics inhibited *C. acnes* growth, reduced inflammation, redness, and acne symptoms, improved wound healing, and enhanced the overall condition of the skin. These findings offer promise for safe, daily acne treatment [140].

A single-arm clinical trial was conducted to investigate the efficacy of heat-treated *Pediococcus acidilactici* LM1013 (HT-LM1013), derived from the Korean traditional fermented alcoholic beverage Makgeolli, as a daily leave-on product for treating acne vulgaris. The investigators found that HT-LM1013 inhibits *C. acnes* biofilm development and reduces lipase activity, decreasing comedone count and sebum production. HT-LM1013 showed promising clinical effects in acne treatment and high patient satisfaction [139].

5.7 Conclusion

Probiotics, prebiotics, and postbiotics are integral components of the microbiome, each playing crucial roles in overall human health (Fig. 5.1). The interplay between these biotics presents a promising potential for managing acne

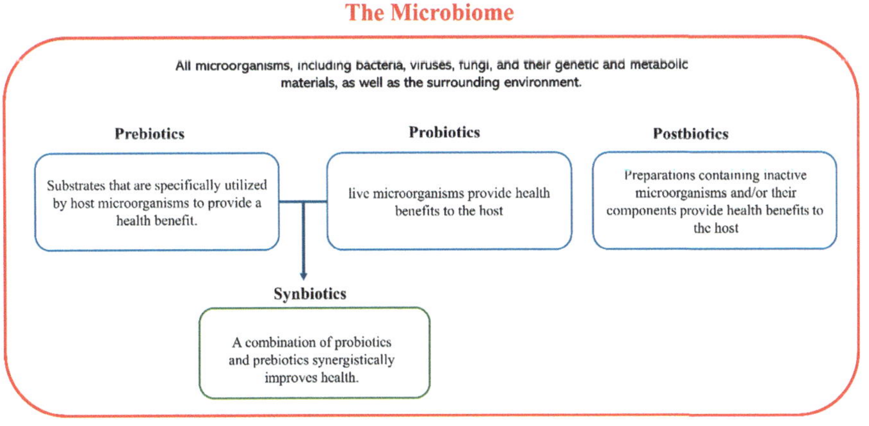

Fig. 5.1 Classification of microbiome biotics: understanding prebiotics, probiotics, postbiotics, and synbiotics

vulgaris. While beneficial to varying degrees, the current acne vulgaris treatment approaches frequently have limitations such as antibiotic resistance, side effects, and incomplete efficacy. Probiotics can modulate gut and skin microbiota, providing a promising alternative or adjuvant treatment to traditional therapies. They directly inhibit the growth of acne-causing bacteria while managing inflammation, thereby improving outcomes for acne patients. Similarly, prebiotics enhance the proliferation of beneficial bacteria, promoting a healthier microbiome and potentially reducing acne severity. Recent findings have shown the potential role of postbiotics in acne treatment, offering probiotic benefits without the risk of live bacteria, and making them a safer option for certain populations. However, further investigations are needed to fully understand the mechanisms and optimize the use of these biotics in acne vulgaris treatment within clinical practice.

In conclusion, integrating probiotics, prebiotics, and postbiotics into acne treatment regimens can significantly improve patient outcomes. This approach aligns with the current understanding of the gut-skin axis and opens new paths for safe and effective acne management strategies.

References

1. Stambler I. A history of life-extensionism in the twentieth century [Undergraduate thesis]. 2011.
2. Hill C, Guarner F, Reid G, Gibson GR, Merenstein DJ, Pot B, et al. Expert consensus document. The International Scientific Association for Probiotics and Prebiotics consensus statement on the scope and appropriate use of the term probiotic. Nat Rev Gastroenterol Hepatol. 2014;11(8):506–14.
3. Fijan S. Microorganisms with claimed probiotic properties: an overview of recent literature. Int J Environ Res Public Health. 2014;11(5):4745–67.
4. Levkovich T, Poutahidis T, Smillie C, Varian BJ, Ibrahim YM, Lakritz JR, et al. Probiotic bacteria induce a "glow of health". PLoS One. 2013;8(1):e53867.
5. Roudsari MR, Karimi R, Sohrabvandi S, Mortazavian AM. Health effects of probiotics on the skin. Crit Rev Food Sci Nutr. 2015;55(9):1219–40.
6. Ahluwalia B, Magnusson MK, Öhman L. Mucosal immune system of the gastrointestinal tract: maintaining balance between the good and the bad. Scand J Gastroenterol. 2017;52(11):1185–93.
7. Iwasaki A, Kelsall BL. Freshly isolated Peyer's patch, but not spleen, dendritic cells produce interleukin 10 and induce the differentiation of T helper type 2 cells. J Exp Med. 1999;190(2):229–39.
8. Friedrich AD, Paz ML, Leoni J, González Maglio DH. Message in a bottle: dialog between intestine and skin modulated by probiotics. Int J Mol Sci. 2017;18(6):1067.
9. Derrien M, Veiga P. Rethinking diet to aid human-microbe symbiosis. Trends Microbiol. 2017;25(2):100–12.
10. Chen B, Li R, Yan N, Chen G, Qian W, Jiang H-L, et al. Astragaloside IV controls collagen reduction in photoaging skin by improving transforming growth factor-β/Smad signaling suppression and inhibiting matrix metalloproteinase-1. Mol Med Rep. 2015;11(5):3344–8.
11. Xia W, Quan T, Hammerberg C, Voorhees JJ, Fisher GJ. A mouse model of skin aging: fragmentation of dermal collagen fibrils and reduced fibroblast spreading due to expression of human matrix metalloproteinase-1. J Dermatol Sci. 2015;78(1):79–82.

12. Jeong JH, Lee CY, Chung DK. Probiotic lactic acid bacteria and skin health. Crit Rev Food Sci Nutr. 2016;56(14):2331–7.
13. Lee DE, Huh C-S, Ra J, Choi I-D, Jeong J-W, Kim S-H, et al. Clinical evidence of effects of Lactobacillus plantarum HY7714 on skin aging: a randomized, double blind, placebo-controlled study. J Microbiol Biotechnol. 2015;25(12):2160–8.
14. Kim HM, Lee DE, Park SD, Kim Y-T, Kim YJ, Jeong JW, et al. Oral administration of lactobacillus plantarum HY7714 protects hairless mouse against ultraviolet B-induced photoaging. J Microbiol Biotechnol. 2014;24(11):1583–91.
15. You G-E, Jung B-J, Kim H-R, Kim H-G, Kim T-R, Chung D-K. Lactobacillus sakei lipoteichoic acid inhibits MMP-1 induced by UVA in normal dermal fibroblasts of human. J Microbiol Biotechnol. 2013;23(10):1357–64.
16. Kober M-M, Bowe WP. The effect of probiotics on immune regulation, acne, and photoaging. Int J Womens Dermatol. 2015;1(2):85–9.
17. Oh S, Kim S-H, Ko Y, Sim J-H, Kim KS, Lee S-H, et al. Effect of bacteriocin produced by Lactococcus sp. HY 449 on skin-inflammatory bacteria. Food Chem Toxicol. 2006;44(4):552–9.
18. Bowe WP, Filip JC, DiRienzo JM, Volgina A, Margolis DJ. Inhibition of propionibacterium acnes by bacteriocin-like inhibitory substances (BLIS) produced by streptococcus salivarius. J Drugs Dermatol. 2006;5(9):868–70.
19. Kang BS, Seo J-G, Lee G-S, Kim J-H, Kim SY, Han YW, et al. Antimicrobial activity of enterocins from enterococcus faecalis SL-5 against propionibacterium acnes, the causative agent in acne vulgaris, and its therapeutic effect. J Microbiol. 2009;47(1):101–9.
20. Lee D-K, Kim M-J, Ham J-W, An H-M, Cha M-K, Lee S-W, et al. In vitro evaluation of antibacterial activities and anti-inflammatory effects of Bifidobacterium spp. addressing acne vulgaris. Arch Pharm Res. 2012;35(6):1065–71.
21. Gueniche A, Benyacoub J, Philippe D, Bastien P, Kusy N, Breton L, et al. Lactobacillus paracasei CNCM I-2116 (ST11) inhibits substance P-induced skin inflammation and accelerates skin barrier function recovery in vitro. Eur J Dermatol. 2010;20(6):731–7.
22. Benyacoub J, Bosco N, Blanchard C, Demont A, Philippe D, Castiel-Higounenc I, et al. Immune modulation property of Lactobacillus paracasei NCC2461 (ST11) strain and impact on skin defences. Benef Microbes. 2014;5(2):129–36.
23. Cosseau C, Devine DA, Dullaghan E, Gardy JL, Chikatamarla A, Gellatly S, et al. The commensal Streptococcus salivarius K12 downregulates the innate immune responses of human epithelial cells and promotes host-microbe homeostasis. Infect Immun. 2008;76(9):4163–75.
24. Espinoza-Monje M, Campos J, Alvarez Villamil E, Jerez A, Dentice Maidana S, Elean M, et al. Characterization of Weissella viridescens UCO-SMC3 as a potential probiotic for the skin: its beneficial role in the pathogenesis of acne vulgaris. Microorganisms. 2021;9(7):1486.
25. Wang Y, Kuo S, Shu M, Yu J, Huang S, Dai A, et al. Staphylococcus epidermidis in the human skin microbiome mediates fermentation to inhibit the growth of Propionibacterium acnes: implications of probiotics in acne vulgaris. Appl Microbiol Biotechnol. 2014;98(1):411–24.
26. Siver RH. Lactobacillus for the control of acne. J Med Soc New Jersey. 1961;59:52–3.
27. Marchetti F, Capizzi R, Tulli A. Efficacy of regulators of the intestinal bacterial flora in the therapy of acne vulgaris. Clin Ter. 1987;122(5):339–43.
28. Volkova LA, Khalif IL, Kabanova IN. Impact of the impaired intestinal microflora on the course of acne vulgaris. Klin Med (Mosk). 2001;79(6):39–41.
29. Kim J, Ko Y, Park Y-K, Kim N-I, Ha W-K, Cho Y. Dietary effect of lactoferrin-enriched fermented milk on skin surface lipid and clinical improvement of acne vulgaris. Nutrition. 2010;26(9):902–9.
30. Manzhalii E, Hornuss D, Stremmel W. Intestinal-borne dermatoses significantly improved by oral application of Escherichia coli Nissle 1917. World J Gastroenterol. 2016;22(23):5415–21.
31. Rahmayani T, Putra IB, Jusuf NK. The effect of oral probiotic on the interleukin-10 serum levels of acne vulgaris. Open Access Maced J Med Sci. 2019;7(19):3249–52.

32. Fabbrocini G, Bertona M, Picazo Ó, Pareja-Galeano H, Monfrecola G, Emanuele E. Supplementation with Lactobacillus rhamnosus SP1 normalises skin expression of genes implicated in insulin signalling and improves adult acne. Benef Microbes. 2016;7(5):625–30.
33. Jung GW, Tse JE, Guiha I, Rao J. Prospective, randomized, open-label trial comparing the safety, efficacy, and tolerability of an acne treatment regimen with and without a probiotic supplement and minocycline in subjects with mild to moderate acne. J Cutan Med Surg. 2013;17(2):114–22.
34. Tolino E, Skroza N, Mambrin A, Bernardini N, Zuber S, Balduzzi V, et al. Novel combination for the treatment of acne differentiated based on gender: a new step towards personalized treatment. G Ital Dermatol Venereol. 2018;153(6):866–71.
35. Rinaldi F, Marotta L, Mascolo A, Amoruso A, Pane M, Giuliani G, et al. Facial acne: a randomized, double-blind, placebo-controlled study on the clinical efficacy of a symbiotic dietary supplement. Dermatol Ther (Heidelb). 2022;12(2):577–89.
36. Eguren C, Navarro-Blasco A, Corral-Forteza M, Reolid-Pérez A, Setó-Torrent N, García-Navarro A, et al. A randomized clinical trial to evaluate the efficacy of an oral probiotic in acne vulgaris. Acta Derm Venereol. 2024;104:adv33206.
37. França K. Topical Probiotics in Dermatological Therapy and Skincare: A Concise Review. Dermatol Ther (Heidelb). 2021;11(1):71–7. https://doi.org/10.1007/s13555-020-00476-7. Epub 2020 Dec 19. PMID: 33340341; PMCID: PMC7859136. URL: https://link.springer.com/article/10.1007/s13555-020-00476-7.
38. Di Marzio L, Cinque B, De Simone C, Cifone MG. Effect of the lactic acid bacterium Streptococcus thermophilus on ceramide levels in human keratinocytes in vitro and stratum corneum in vivo. J Invest Dermatol. 1999;113(1):98–106.
39. Ho VPY, Ma E, Liew HM, Ng MSY, Koh MJA. Comparing the potential for irritation of a ceramide-based moisturizer with a urea-based moisturizer for pediatric atopic dermatitis. Dermatol Ther (Heidelb). 2020;10(4):807–13.
40. Di Marzio L, Cinque B, Cupelli F, De Simone C, Cifone MG, Giuliani M. Increase of skin-ceramide levels in aged subjects following a short-term topical application of bacterial sphingomyelinase from Streptococcus thermophilus. Int J Immunopathol Pharmacol. 2008;21(1):137–43.
41. Di Marzio L, Centi C, Cinque B, Masci S, Giuliani M, Arcieri A, et al. Effect of the lactic acid bacterium Streptococcus thermophilus on stratum corneum ceramide levels and signs and symptoms of atopic dermatitis patients. Exp Dermatol. 2003;12(5):615–20.
42. Pavicic T, Wollenweber U, Farwick M, Korting HC. Anti-microbial and -inflammatory activity and efficacy of phytosphingosine: an in vitro and in vivo study addressing acne vulgaris. Int J Cosmet Sci. 2007;29(3):181–90.
43. Muizzuddin N, Maher W, Sullivan M, Schnittger S, Mammone T. Physiological effect of a probiotic on skin. J Cosmet Sci. 2012;63(6):385–95.
44. Sathikulpakdee S, Kanokrungsee S, Vitheejongjaroen P, Kamanamool N, Udompataikul M, Taweechotipatr M. Efficacy of probiotic-derived lotion from Lactobacillus paracasei MSMC 39-1 in mild to moderate acne vulgaris, randomized controlled trial. J Cosmet Dermatol. 2022;21(10):5092–7.
45. Gibson GR, Roberfroid MB. Dietary modulation of the human colonic microbiota: introducing the concept of prebiotics. J Nutr. 1995;125(6):1401–12.
46. Gibson GR, Hutkins R, Sanders ME, Prescott SL, Reimer RA, Salminen SJ, et al. Expert consensus document: The International Scientific Association for Probiotics and Prebiotics (ISAPP) consensus statement on the definition and scope of prebiotics. Nat Rev Gastroenterol Hepatol. 2017;14(8):491–502.
47. Panesar PS, Kumari S, Panesar R. Biotechnological approaches for the production of prebiotics and their potential applications. Crit Rev Biotechnol. 2013;33(4):345–64.
48. Al-Sheraji SH, Ismail A, Manap MY, Mustafa S, Yusof RM, Hassan FA. Prebiotics as functional foods: a review. J Funct Foods. 2013;5(4):1542–53.

49. Varzakas T, Kandylis P, Dimitrellou D, Salamoura C, Zakynthinos G, Proestos C. Innovative and fortified food: Probiotics, prebiotics, GMOs, and superfood. In: Preparation and processing of religious and cultural foods. Elsevier; 2018. p. 67–129.
50. Louis P, Flint HJ, Michel C. How to manipulate the microbiota: prebiotics. Adv Exp Med Biol. 2016;902:119–42.
51. Scott KP, Martin JC, Duncan SH, Flint HJ. Prebiotic stimulation of human colonic butyrate-producing bacteria and bifidobacteria, in vitro. FEMS Microbiol Ecol. 2014;87(1):30–40.
52. Macfarlane GT, Steed H, Macfarlane S. Bacterial metabolism and health-related effects of galacto-oligosaccharides and other prebiotics. J Appl Microbiol. 2008;104(2):305–44.
53. Gibson GR, Scott KP, Rastall RA, Tuohy KM, Hotchkiss A, Dubert-Ferrandon A, et al. Dietary prebiotics: current status and new definition. Food Sci Technol Bull Funct Foods. 2010;7(1):1–19.
54. Whelan K. Mechanisms and effectiveness of prebiotics in modifying the gastrointestinal microbiota for the management of digestive disorders. Proc Nutr Soc. 2013;72(3):288–98.
55. Johnson CR, Thavarajah D, Combs GF, Thavarajah P. Lentil (Lens culinaris L.): a prebiotic-rich whole food legume. Food Res Int. 2013;51(1):107–13.
56. Fuentes-Zaragoza E, Sánchez-Zapata E, Sendra E, Sayas E, Navarro C, Fernández-López J, et al. Resistant starch as prebiotic: a review. Starch/Stärke. 2011;63(7):406–15.
57. Ze X, Duncan SH, Louis P, Flint HJ. Ruminococcus bromii is a keystone species for the degradation of resistant starch in the human colon. ISME J. 2012;6(8):1535–43.
58. Walker AW, Ince J, Duncan SH, Webster LM, Holtrop G, Ze X, et al. Dominant and diet-responsive groups of bacteria within the human colonic microbiota. ISME J. 2011;5(2):220–30.
59. Costabile A, Fava F, Röytiö H, Forssten SD, Olli K, Klievink J, et al. Impact of polydextrose on the faecal microbiota: a double-blind, crossover, placebo-controlled feeding study in healthy human subjects. Br J Nutr. 2012;108(3):471–81.
60. Gullón B, Gómez B, Martínez-Sabajanes M, Yáñez R, Parajó JC, Alonso JL. Pectic oligosaccharides: manufacture and functional properties. Trends Food Sci Technol. 2013;30(2):153–61.
61. Yoo H-D, Kim D, Paek S-H. Plant cell wall polysaccharides as potential resources for the development of novel prebiotics. Biomol Ther (Seoul). 2012;20(4):371–9.
62. Tzounis X, Rodriguez-Mateos A, Vulevic J, Gibson GR, Kwik-Uribe C, Spencer JPE. Prebiotic evaluation of cocoa-derived flavanols in healthy humans by using a randomized, controlled, double-blind, crossover intervention study. Am J Clin Nutr. 2011;93(1):62–72.
63. Lolou V, Panayiotidis MI. Functional role of probiotics and prebiotics on skin health and disease. Fermentation. 2019;5(2):41.
64. Grajek W, Olejnik A, Sip A. Probiotics, prebiotics and antioxidants as functional foods. Acta Biochim Pol. 2005;52(3):665–71.
65. Schley PD, Field CJ. The immune-enhancing effects of dietary fibres and prebiotics. Br J Nutr. 2002;87(Suppl 2):S221–30.
66. Van den Abbeele P, Venema K, Van de Wiele T, Verstraete W, Possemiers S. Different human gut models reveal the distinct fermentation patterns of Arabinoxylan versus inulin. J Agric Food Chem. 2013;61(41):9819–27.
67. Sivieri K, Morales MLV, Saad SMI, Adorno MAT, Sakamoto IK, Rossi EA. Prebiotic effect of fructooligosaccharide in the simulator of the human intestinal microbial ecosystem (SHIME® model). J Med Food. 2014;17(8):894–901.
68. Bruzzese E, Volpicelli M, Salvini F, Bisceglia M, Lionetti P, Cinquetti M, et al. Early administration of gos/fos prevents intestinal and respiratory infections in infants. J Pediatr Gastroenterol Nutr. 2006;42(5):E95.
69. Scholtens PAMJ, Alliet P, Raes M, Alles MS, Kroes H, Boehm G, et al. Fecal secretory immunoglobulin A is increased in healthy infants who receive a formula with short-chain galacto-oligosaccharides and long-chain fructo-oligosaccharides. J Nutr. 2008;138(6):1141–7.
70. Al-Ghazzewi FH, Tester RF. Effect of konjac glucomannan hydrolysates and probiotics on the growth of the skin bacterium propionibacterium acnes in vitro. Int J Cosmet Sci. 2010;32(2):139–42.

71. Elamir AA, Tester RF, Al-Ghazzewi FH, Kaal HY, Ghalbon AA, Elmegrahai NA, et al. Effects of konjac glucomannan hydrolysates on the gut microflora of mice. Nutr Food Sci. 2008;38(5):422–9.
72. Al-Ghazzewi FH, Tester RF. Efficacy of cellulase and mannanase hydrolysates of konjac glucomannan to promote the growth of lactic acid bacteria. J Sci Food Agric. 2012;92(11):2394–6.
73. Al-Ghazzewi FH, Khanna S, Tester RF, Piggott J. The potential use of hydrolysed konjac glucomannan as a prebiotic. J Sci Food Agric. 2007;87(9):1758–66.
74. Geier MS, Butler RN, Howarth GS. Probiotics, prebiotics and synbiotics: a role in chemoprevention for colorectal cancer? Cancer Biol Ther. 2006;5(10):1265–9.
75. Al-Ghazzewi FH, Tester RF. Impact of prebiotics and probiotics on skin health. Benef Microbes. 2014;5(2):99–107. https://doi.org/10.3920/BM2013.0040. PMID: 24583611. URL: https://brill.com/view/journals/bm/5/2/article-p99_99.xml.
76. Tester R, Al-Ghazzewi F, Shen N, Chen Z, Chen F, Yang J, et al. The use of konjac glucomannan hydrolysates to recover healthy microbiota in infected vaginas treated with an antifungal agent. Benef Microbes. 2012;3(1):61–6.
77. Sutherland A, Tester R, Al-Ghazzewi F. Glucomannan hydrolysate (GMH) inhibition of Candida albicans growth in the presence of Lactobacillus and Lactococcus species. Microb Ecol Health Dis. 2008;20(3):127–34.
78. Moro G, Arslanoglu S, Stahl B, Jelinek J, Wahn U, Boehm G. A mixture of prebiotic oligosaccharides reduces the incidence of atopic dermatitis during the first six months of age. Arch Dis Child. 2006;91(10):814–9.
79. Lindsay JO, Whelan K, Stagg AJ, Gobin P, Al-Hassi HO, Rayment N, et al. Clinical, microbiological, and immunological effects of fructo-oligosaccharide in patients with Crohn's disease. Gut. 2006;55(3):348–55.
80. Welters CFM, Heineman E, Thunnissen FBJM, van den Bogaard AEJM, Soeters PB, Baeten CGMI. Effect of dietary inulin supplementation on inflammation of pouch mucosa in patients with an ileal pouch-anal anastomosis. Dis Colon Rectum. 2002;45(5):621–7.
81. Onishi N, Kawamoto S, Ueda K, Yamanaka Y, Katayama A, Suzuki H, et al. Dietary pulverized konjac glucomannan prevents the development of allergic rhinitis-like symptoms and IgE response in mice. Biosci Biotechnol Biochem. 2007;71(10):2551–6.
82. Suzuki H, Oomizu S, Yanase Y, Onishi N, Uchida K, Mihara S, et al. Hydrolyzed Konjac glucomannan suppresses IgE production in mice B cells. Int Arch Allergy Immunol. 2010;152(2):122–30.
83. Pérez-Conesa D, López G, Abellán P, Ros G. Bioavailability of calcium, magnesium and phosphorus in rats fed probiotic, prebiotic and synbiotic powder follow-up infant formulas and their effect on physiological and nutritional parameters. J Sci Food Agric. 2006;86(14):2327–36.
84. Shakeri H, Hadaegh H, Abedi F, Tajabadi-Ebrahimi M, Mazroii N, Ghandi Y, et al. Consumption of synbiotic bread decreases triacylglycerol and VLDL levels while increasing HDL levels in serum from patients with type-2 diabetes. Lipids. 2014;49(7):695–701.
85. Parnell JA, Reimer RA. Weight loss during oligofructose supplementation is associated with decreased ghrelin and increased peptide YY in overweight and obese adults. Am J Clin Nutr. 2009;89(6):1751–9.
86. Miyazaki K, Masuoka N, Kano M, Iizuka R. Bifidobacterium fermented milk and galacto-oligosaccharides lead to improved skin health by decreasing phenols production by gut microbiota. Benef Microbes. 2014;5(2):121–8.
87. Kawakami K, Marino I, Asahara T, Kato I, Onoue M. Dietary galacto-oligosaccharides mixture can suppress serum phenol and p-cresol levels in rats fed tyrosine diet. J Nutr Sci Vitaminol. 2005;51(3):182–6.
88. Kano M, Masuoka N, Kaga C, Sugimoto S, Iizuka R, Manabe K, et al. Consecutive intake of fermented milk containing bifidobacterium breve Strain Yakult and Galacto-oligosaccharides benefits skin condition in healthy adult women. Biosci Microbiota Food Health. 2013;32(1):33–9.

89. Hong K-B, Jeong M, Han KS, Hwan Kim J, Park Y, Suh HJ. Photoprotective effects of galacto-oligosaccharide and/or Bifidobacterium longum supplementation against skin damage induced by ultraviolet irradiation in hairless mice. Int J Food Sci Nutr. 2015;66(8):923–30.
90. Akiyama H, Oono T, Huh WK, Yamasaki O, Akagi Y, Uemura H, et al. Actions of gluco-oligosaccharide against Staphylococcus aureus. J Dermatol. 2002;29(9):580–6.
91. Grüber C, van Stuijvenberg M, Mosca F, Moro G, Chirico G, Braegger CP, et al. Reduced occurrence of early atopic dermatitis because of immunoactive prebiotics among low-atopy-risk infants. J Allergy Clin Immunol. 2010;126(4):791–7.
92. Zareie E, Mansouri P, Hosseini H, Sadeghpour O, Shirbeigi L, Hejazi S, et al. Effect of oral administration of triphala, a polyphenol-rich prebiotic, on scalp sebum in patients with scalp seborrhea a randomized clinical trial. J Dermatolog Treat. 2022;33(2):1011–6.
93. Pandey KR, Naik SR, Vakil BV. Probiotics, prebiotics and synbiotics—a review. J Food Sci Technol. 2015;52(12):7577–87.
94. Al-Ghazzewi FH, Tester RF. Impact of prebiotics and probiotics on skin health. Benef Microbes. 2014;5(2):99–107.
95. Kazandjieva J, Dimitrova J, Sankeva M, Yankov D, Bocheva V, Kircheva K, et al. Efficacy of a retinoid complex plus anti-inflammatory component cream alone or in combination with prebiotic food supplement in adult acne: a randomized, assessor-blinded, parallel-group, multicenter trial on 184 women. J Cosmet Dermatol. 2022;21(11):5716–22.
96. Dall'Oglio F, Milani M, Micali G. Effects of oral supplementation with FOS and GOS prebiotics in women with adult acne: the "S.O. Sweet" study: a proof-of-concept pilot trial. Clin Cosmet Investig Dermatol. 2018;11:445–9.
97. Fooks LJ, Gibson GR. Probiotics as modulators of the gut flora. Br J Nutr. 2002;88(Suppl 1):S39–49.
98. Su P, Henriksson A, Mitchell H. Prebiotics enhance survival and prolong the retention period of specific probiotic inocula in an in vivo murine model. J Appl Microbiol. 2007;103(6):2392–400.
99. Sekhon BS, Jairath S. Prebiotics, probiotics and synbiotics: an overview. J Pharm Educ Res. 2010;1:13–36.
100. Markowiak P, Śliżewska K. Effects of probiotics, prebiotics, and synbiotics on human health. Nutrients. 2017;9(9):1021.
101. Tajadadi Ebrahimi M, Bahmani F, Shakeri H, Hadaegh H, Hijijafari M, Abedi F, et al. Effects of daily consumption of synbiotic bread on insulin metabolism and serum high-sensitivity C-reactive protein among diabetic patients: a double-blind, randomized, controlled clinical trial. Ann Nutr Metab. 2014;65(1):34–41.
102. Sergeev IN, Aljutaily T, Walton G, Huarte E. Effects of synbiotic supplement on human gut microbiota, body composition and weight loss in obesity. Nutrients. 2020;12(1):222.
103. Jiang H, Cai M, Shen B, Wang Q, Zhang T, Zhou X. Synbiotics and gut microbiota: new perspectives in the treatment of type 2 diabetes mellitus. Food Secur. 2022;11(16):2438.
104. Phavichitr N, Wang S, Chomto S, Tantibhaedhyangkul R, Kakourou A, Intarakhao S, et al. Impact of synbiotics on gut microbiota during early life: a randomized, double-blind study. Sci Rep. 2021;11(1):3534.
105. Liu F, Li P, Chen M, Luo Y, Prabhakar M, Zheng H, et al. Fructooligosaccharide (FOS) and galactooligosaccharide (GOS) increase bifidobacterium but reduce butyrate producing bacteria with adverse glycemic metabolism in healthy young population. Sci Rep. 2017;7(1):11789.
106. Sanchez M, Darimont C, Drapeau V, Emady-Azar S, Lepage M, Rezzonico E, et al. Effect of Lactobacillus rhamnosus CGMCC1.3724 supplementation on weight loss and maintenance in obese men and women. Br J Nutr. 2014;111(8):1507–19.
107. Simon E, Călinoiu LF, Mitrea L, Vodnar DC. Probiotics, prebiotics, and synbiotics: implications and beneficial effects against irritable bowel syndrome. Nutrients. 2021;13(6):2112.
108. Ritchie ML, Romanuk TN. A meta-analysis of probiotic efficacy for gastrointestinal diseases. PLoS One. 2012;7(4):e34938.

109. Ford AC, Harris LA, Lacy BE, Quigley EMM, Moayyedi P. Systematic review with meta-analysis: the efficacy of prebiotics, probiotics, synbiotics and antibiotics in irritable bowel syndrome. Aliment Pharmacol Ther. 2018;48(10):1044–60.
110. Ouwehand AC, Salminen S, Isolauri E. Probiotics: an overview of beneficial effects. Antonie Van Leeuwenhoek. 2002;82(1–4):279–89.
111. Bojar RA, Holland KT. The human cutaneous microflora and factors controlling colonisation. World J Microbiol Biotechnol. 2002;18:889–903.
112. Tester RF, Al-Ghazzewi FH. Mannans and health, with a special focus on glucomannans. Food Res Int. 2013;50(1):384–91.
113. Taverniti V, Guglielmetti S. The immunomodulatory properties of probiotic microorganisms beyond their viability (ghost probiotics: proposal of paraprobiotic concept). Genes Nutr. 2011;6(3):261–74.
114. Nataraj BH, Ali SA, Behare PV, Yadav H. Postbiotics-parabiotics: the new horizons in microbial biotherapy and functional foods. Microb Cell Factories. 2020;19(1):168.
115. Wilcox H, Carr C, Seney S, Reid G, Burton JP. Expired probiotics: what is really in your cabinet? FEMS Microbes. 2020;1(1):xtaa007.
116. Jorjão AL, Oliveira FE, Leão MVP. Live and heat-killed lactobacillus rhamnosus ATCC 7469 may induce modulatory cytokines profiles on macrophages RAW 264.7. ScientificWorldJournal. 2015;2015:716749.
117. Chuang L, Wu K-G, Pai C, Hsieh P-S, Tsai J-J, Yen J-H, et al. Heat-killed cells of lactobacilli skew the immune response toward T helper 1 polarization in mouse splenocytes and dendritic cell-treated T cells. J Agric Food Chem. 2007;55(26):11080–6.
118. Salminen S, Collado MC, Endo A, Hill C, Lebeer S, Quigley EMM, et al. The International Scientific Association of Probiotics and Prebiotics (ISAPP) consensus statement on the definition and scope of postbiotics. Nat Rev Gastroenterol Hepatol. 2021;18(9):649–67.
119. Tsilingiri K, Rescigno M. Postbiotics: what else? Benef Microbes. 2013;4(1):101–7.
120. Wegh CAM, Geerlings SY, Knol J, Roeselers G, Belzer C. Postbiotics and their potential applications in early life nutrition and beyond. Int J Mol Sci. 2019;20(19):4673.
121. de Almada CN, Almada CN, Martinez RCR, Sant'Ana AS. Paraprobiotics: evidences on their ability to modify biological responses, inactivation methods and perspectives on their application in foods. Trends Food Sci Technol. 2016;58:96–114.
122. Żółkiewicz J, Marzec A, Ruszczyński M, Feleszko W. Postbiotics-A step beyond pre- and probiotics. Nutrients. 2020;12(8):2189.
123. Klemashevich C, Wu C, Howsmon D, Alaniz RC, Lee K, Jayaraman A. Rational identification of diet-derived postbiotics for improving intestinal microbiota function. Curr Opin Biotechnol. 2014;26:85–90.
124. Martyniak A, Medyńska-Przęczek A, Wędrychowicz A, Skoczeń S, Tomasik PJ. Prebiotics, probiotics, synbiotics, paraprobiotics and postbiotic compounds in IBD. Biomol Ther. 2021;11(12):1903.
125. Imperial ICVJ, Ibana JA. Addressing the antibiotic resistance problem with probiotics: reducing the risk of its double-edged sword effect. Front Microbiol. 2016;7:1983.
126. Inoue Y, Kambara T, Murata N, Komori-Yamaguchi J, Matsukura S, Takahashi Y, et al. Effects of oral administration of lactobacillus acidophilus L-92 on the symptoms and serum cytokines of atopic dermatitis in Japanese adults: a double-blind, randomized. Clinical Trial Int Arch Allergy Immunol. 2014;165(4):247–54.
127. Catic T, Pehlivanovic B, Pljakic N, Balicevac A. The moisturizing efficacy of a proprietary dermo-cosmetic product (CLS02021) versus placebo in a 4-week application period. Med Arch. 2022;76(2):108–14.
128. da Silva Vale A, de Melo Pereira GV, de Oliveira AC, de Carvalho Neto DP, Herrmann LW, Karp SG, et al. Production, formulation, and application of postbiotics in the treatment of skin conditions. Fermentation. 2023;9(3):264.
129. Rinaldi F, Trink A, Pinto D. Efficacy of postbiotics in a PRP-like cosmetic product for the treatment of alopecia area celsi: a randomized double-blinded parallel-group study. Dermatol Ther (Heidelb). 2020;10(3):483–93.

130. Rong J, Shan C, Liu S, Zheng H, Liu C, Liu M, et al. Skin resistance to UVB-induced oxidative stress and hyperpigmentation by the topical use of lactobacillus helveticus NS8-fermented milk supernatant. J Appl Microbiol. 2017;123(2):511–23.
131. Golkar N, Ashoori Y, Heidari R, Omidifar N, Abootalebi SN, Mohkam M, et al. A novel effective formulation of bioactive compounds for wound healing: preparation, in vivo characterization, and comparison of various postbiotics cold creams in a rat model. Evid Based Complement Alternat Med. 2021;2021:8577116.
132. Lee S-H, Yoon J-M, Kim Y-H, Jeong D-G, Park S, Kang D-J. Therapeutic effect of tyndallized lactobacillus rhamnosus IDCC 3201 on atopic dermatitis mediated by down-regulation of immunoglobulin E in NC/Nga mice. Microbiol Immunol. 2016;60(7):468–76.
133. Choi E-J, Iwasa M, Han K-I, Kim W-J, Tang Y, Hwang YJ, et al. Heat-killed enterococcus faecalis EF-2001 ameliorates atopic dermatitis in a murine model. Nutrients. 2016;8(3):146.
134. Im A-R, Lee B, Kang D-J, Chae S. Skin moisturizing and antiphotodamage effects of tyndallized lactobacillus acidophilus IDCC 3302. J Med Food. 2018;21(10):1016–23.
135. Ogawa M, Saiki A, Matsui Y, Tsuchimoto N, Nakakita Y, Takata Y, et al. Effects of oral intake of heat-killed Lactobacillus brevis SBC8803 (SBL88TM) on dry skin conditions: a randomized, double-blind, placebo-controlled study. Exp Ther Med. 2016;12(6):3863–72.
136. Chung H-J, Lee H, Kim M, Lee JW, Saeed M, Lee H, et al. Development and metabolic profiling of a postbiotic complex exhibiting antibacterial activity against skin microorganisms and anti-inflammatory effect on human keratinocytes. Food Sci Biotechnol. 2022;31(10):1325–34.
137. Majeed M, Majeed S, Nagabhushanam K, Lawrence L, Arumugam S, Mundkur L. Skin protective activity of lactosporin-the extracellular metabolite from bacillus coagulans MTCC 5856. Cosmetics. 2020;7(4):76.
138. Majeed M, Majeed S, Nagabhushanam K, Mundkur L, Rajalakshmi H, Shah K, et al. Novel topical application of a postbiotic, lactosporin®, in mild to moderate acne: a randomized, comparative clinical study to evaluate its efficacy, tolerability and safety. Cosmetics. 2020;7(3):70.
139. Bae W-Y, Jung W-H, Lee YJ, Shin SL, An Y-K, Kim T-R, et al. Heat-treated Pediococcus acidilactici LM1013-mediated inhibition of biofilm formation by Cutibacterium acnes and its application in acne vulgaris: a single-arm clinical trial. J Cosmet Dermatol. 2023;22(11):3125–34.
140. Ho H-H, Chen C-W, Yi T-H, Huang Y-F, Kuo Y-W, Lin J-H, et al. Novel application of a Co-Fermented postbiotics of TYCA06/AP-32/CP-9/collagen in the improvement of acne vulgaris—a randomized clinical study of efficacy evaluation. J Cosmet Dermatol. 2022;21(11):6249–60.
141. Cui H, Guo C, Wang Q, Feng C, Duan Z. A pilot study on the efficacy of topical lotion containing anti-acne postbiotic in subjects with mild to moderate acne. Front Med (Lausanne). 2022;9:1064460.
142. Cui H, Feng C, Guo C, Duan Z. Development of novel topical anti-acne cream containing postbiotics for mild-to-moderate acne: an observational study to evaluate its efficacy. Indian J Dermatol. 2022;67(6):667–73.
143. Kang Y-K, Chen L-T, Ryu M-H, Oh D-Y, Oh SC, Chung HC, et al. Nivolumab plus chemotherapy versus placebo plus chemotherapy in patients with HER2-negative, untreated, unresectable advanced or recurrent gastric or gastro-oesophageal junction cancer (ATTRACTION-4): a randomised, multicentre, double-blind, placebo-controlled, phase 3 trial. Lancet Oncol. 2022;23(2):234–47.
144. Han HS, Shin SH, Choi B-Y, Koo N, Lim S, Son D, et al. A split face study on the effect of an anti-acne product containing fermentation products of Enterococcus faecalis CBT SL-5 on skin microbiome modification and acne improvement. J Microbiol. 2022;60(5):488–95.

The Effect of Vitamins, and Minerals on Acne Vulgaris Treatment

6

Nereen A. Almosilhy, Amr S. Ghattas,
and Esraa M. AlEdani

Contents

The original version of the chapter has been revised. A correction to this chapter can be found at https://doi.org/10.1007/978-3-031-83677-0_9

N. A. Almosilhy (✉)
Department of Pharmacology and Toxicology, Faculty of Pharmacy, Tanta University, Tanta, Egypt

A. S. Ghattas
Faculty of Medicine, Cairo University, Giza, Egypt

E. M. AlEdani
Basra Medical College, Basrah, Iraq

E. M. AlEdani, H. I. Maibach (eds.), *Nutrition and Acne Vulgaris*, Updates in Clinical Dermatology, https://doi.org/10.1007/978-3-031-83677-0_6

6.1 Vitamins Overview

Recent research reveals that the combination of a proper diet and vitamin supplementation with standard drug therapy may dramatically improve acne lesions and enhance patient satisfaction.

Vitamins are a class of micronutrients (or collections of molecules) that are essential for various physiological functions. Since the body cannot synthesize most vitamins, they must be obtained from external sources such as diet, supplements, fortified foods, and, in the case of vitamins D and K, from sunlight and gut flora, respectively. Each vitamin serves specific crucial roles in the human body. For instance, vitamin A is essential for vision, immune function and reproduction, and regulates cell growth and differentiation, while the B-complex vitamins act as enzyme precursors or cofactors in energy metabolism, brain function, red blood cell production, and overall cell health. Vitamin D functions as a prohormone that maintains calcium and phosphorus homeostasis, and vitamins C and E primarily serve as free radical scavengers and antioxidants. Vitamins have been found to play a crucial role in the management of acne vulgaris. For example, vitamin A and D reduce inflammation and sebum production, while Vitamin E and C provide antioxidant protection. Vitamin B3 (niacinamide) also helps control sebum and inflammation, but excessive Vitamin B12 may worsen acne symptoms. While vitamin supplements can be beneficial, it is important to be cautious of hypervitaminosis, particularly with fat-soluble vitamins A, D, E, and K, which can accumulate in the body and become toxic over time, leading to potential health risks. In contrast, vitamins B complex and C are water-soluble and are readily excreted through urine; therefore, consistent intake is necessary, even though toxicity from these vitamins is unlikely.

6.2 Vitamin A

Vitamin A comprises a group of fat-soluble retinoids, including retinal, retinol, and retinyl esters, which are essential for survival due to their role in regulating and supporting vision, immunity, reproduction, bone development, skin health, cell growth and differentiation. Vitamin A can be sourced from plants as carotenoids (provitamin A) or from animals as retinol and related derivatives. Although retinol and retinyl esters are typically prevalent in the human body, the oxidized derivatives 11-cis-retinal and all-trans-retinoic acid (ATRA) are the primary bioactive molecules [1]. In the intestinal lumen, dietary retinol is absorbed directly into enterocytes. However, for the absorption of unesterified retinol, and dietary retinyl esters must undergo enzymatic hydrolysis either within the lumen or at the enterocyte brush border. Unlike dietary retinoids, proretinoid carotenoids (e.g., β-carotene) can either be converted to retinal within enterocytes or absorbed in their original form [2].

6.2.1 Vitamin A: Essential Retinoids for Acne Vulgaris Treatment

The skin is particularly sensitive to retinoids due to their ability to bind to retinoic acid receptors in the cell nuclei of both the epidermis and dermis layers [3]. Retinoic acid is considered the most effective form for treating acne because it targets several key etiological factors, including the reduction of sebum excretion, shrinkage of sebaceous glands, decreased keratinization, regulation of cell proliferation, reduction in the number of *Propionibacterium acnes* (*P. acnes*), and inhibition of comedogenesis. Additionally, retinoic acid exhibits anti-inflammatory and immunomodulatory effects by decreasing the expression of Toll-Like Receptor 2 (TLR-2) and reducing the inflammatory cytokine response, along with antineoplastic properties. These mechanisms make both topical and oral retinoic acid effective in treating acne and beneficial for other skin conditions, such as improving scar appearance, treating dyspigmentation, and acting as an anti-aging agent [4]. Isotretinoin, a 13-cis-retinoic acid derivative of vitamin A, was FDA-approved in 1982 as an oral medication for severe, treatment-resistant acne. It reduces sebaceous gland activity, normalizes keratinization, and alleviates inflammation. Its off-label uses include cutaneous T-cell lymphomas, neuroblastoma, and certain skin cancers, as well as other dermatological conditions such as rosacea, folliculitis, and pyoderma faciale. While oral isotretinoin does not have direct antimicrobial effects, it significantly reduces the size of pilosebaceous ducts, and decreases the presence of *P. acnes* colonization [4, 5].

6.2.2 Dosage and Safety Considerations for Isotretinoin in Acne Treatment

Conventionally, oral isotretinoin is prescribed twice daily at a dose ranging from 0.5 to 1 mg/kg. If the standard dose is not well tolerated, due to its commonly associated adverse effects, including extreme skin and mucosal dryness (lips, skin, eyes, nose, genitals), eczema, increased sweating, nosebleeds, and facial erythema, it can be reduced, with the option to increase it back to 1 mg/kg if needed. The typical treatment course lasts 4–6 months, depending on the frequency of use. If acne has improved by over 90% from baseline, the treatment should be discontinued and may be restarted after 30 to 60 days if necessary [4]. A systematic review by Sadeghzadeh-Bazargan et al. [7] recommended reduced doses of isotretinoin (between 0.1 and 1 mg/kg, particularly at the lower end of this range) compared to standard dosing protocols in acne vulgaris treatment [7]. Isotretinoin poses a 20–35% risk of severe congenital defects, including craniofacial, neurological, cardiovascular, and thymic abnormalities, in exposed infants, even with short-term exposure at all therapeutic doses. This risk arises from its ability to induce apoptosis and cell cycle arrest in sebocytes, contributing to its teratogenic effects affecting both fertile females and males. Therefore, strict pregnancy prevention programs are mandatory, such as the iPLEDGE program, a U.S. Food and Drug Administration (FDA)-required Risk Evaluation and Mitigation Strategy (REMS), to guarantee that the therapeutic advantages of isotretinoin outweigh its potential risks throughout the treatment course [4, 6].

6.3 Vitamin D

Vitamin D is a fat-soluble vitamin naturally present in a limited range of foods, including egg yolks, oily fish, and liver. However, the primary source of vitamin D is dermal synthesis in response to ultraviolet-B (UVB) radiation, which accounts for approximately 90% of the body's vitamin D content [8]. Upon exposure to UVB, 7-dehydrocholesterol in the epidermal cells is converted to pre-vitamin D3, a biologically inactive form, which undergoes hydroxylation in the liver to form 25-hydroxyvitamin D [25(OH)D], also known as calcidiol. Further hydroxylation occurs in the kidneys, producing the active form, 1,25-dihydroxyvitamin D [1,25(OH)2D], or calcitriol, which is the most biologically active form of vitamin D [9].

Vitamin D plays a critical role in the human body by influencing serum calcium homeostasis and regulating cell division, proliferation, and apoptosis through both paracrine and autocrine mechanisms. It has been found to have a role in both innate and adaptive immune responses, acting as an immunomodulator in various autoimmune diseases, including lupus erythematosus, vitiligo, multiple sclerosis, alopecia, inflammatory bowel disease, psoriasis, and atopic dermatitis [10–14].

6.3.1 Rationale for Vitamin D Use in Acne Vulgaris Treatment

Human sebocytes possess vitamin D receptors that may influence lipid synthesis, suggesting a potential role in regulating sebum production, skin barrier function, and inflammation. An *in vitro* experiment found that in these cells, calcitriol, the active form of vitamin D, inhibits sebocyte growth and differentiation in a dose-dependent manner, thereby regulating sebum production [15, 16]. Additionally, vitamin D reduces inflammation in acne patients through multiple mechanisms, including the activation of TLR2, which initiates innate immune responses with antibacterial effects, inhibition of *P. acnes*-induced IL-17, and the downregulation of inflammatory mediators and cytokines such as Matrix Metalloproteinase-9 (MMP-9), IL-6, and IL-8 [16–19]. Thus, vitamin D potentially alleviates acne vulgaris by reducing sebum production, exerting antibacterial effects, and mitigating inflammation.

6.3.2 Clinical Evidence on Vitamin D Efficacy in Acne Vulgaris Treatment

Several clinical studies show mixed evidence between vitamin D and acne symptoms, but many have demonstrated an inverse association between serum vitamin D levels and acne vulgaris [17, 20–22]. For instance, a cross-sectional study involving 68 acne patients, and 50 healthy controls found that serum 25-hydroxyvitamin D levels were significantly lower in the acne patient group [17]. However, other investigations, including a large cross-sectional study of 714 adolescents and young adults that controlled confounding variables, failed to confirm these findings [23, 24]. Nevertheless, a comprehensive review and meta-analysis by Wang et al. [25], which included 918 acne patients and 814 controls, concluded that acne patients had lower serum 25(OH)D levels.

Moreover, a prospective, randomized controlled trial (RCT) involving 100 acne patients revealed that four out of five patients with severe acne were deficient in vitamin D, suggesting a negative association between vitamin D levels and acne severity. Notably, the trial also found that patients who received a daily dose of alfacalcidol (0.25 μg) for 3 months showed significant improvement in acne severity compared to the placebo group, highlighting the potential beneficial role of vitamin D in acne management and treatment, but further research is needed [12]. In another double-blinded split-face trial conducted on 40 acne patients, calcipotriol (a topical synthetic vitamin D2) was applied to one side of the face, while adapalene (a synthetic retinoid) was applied to the other side over 2 months. The results indicated a decrease in the number of comedones and total acne lesions on both sides, with no statistically significant difference in clinical outcomes. However, histopathological findings revealed a median reduction of 100% in the total inflammatory score on the calcipotriol-treated side compared to a 66.7% reduction on the adapalene-treated side, indicating that calcipotriol may have a more potent anti-inflammatory effect in the treatment of acne vulgaris [26]. Vitamin D has a safe intake limit, similar to other fat-soluble vitamins; hence, a daily intake of 10,000 to 40,000 IU is considered toxic as it disrupts calcium homeostasis [27].

6.4 Vitamin C

Vitamin C, also referred to as L-ascorbic acid, is a water-soluble vitamin that comprises several molecules, including magnesium ascorbyl phosphate, ascorbyl phosphate, sodium calcium ascorbate, and sodium ascorbate [28, 29]. While most species can synthesize vitamin C, higher-order primates, including humans, cannot. As a result, vitamin C is an essential dietary nutrient for humans, obtained primarily through fruits and vegetables [30]. Insufficient intake of vitamin C can lead to scurvy, a disease characterized by symptoms such as fatigue, swollen gums, capillary fragility, and bleeding [31, 32]. Vitamin C is a potent antioxidant essential for collagen synthesis, L-carnitine production, certain neurotransmitter synthesis, and protein metabolism [28, 33, 34]. It helps absorb non-heme iron, promotes immune function, and may also reduce the risk of cancer and cardiovascular disease [28, 33, 35–37].

Vitamin C is highly concentrated in the skin, indicating its significant role in skin function, particularly in the synthesis of dermal collagen, and providing protection against photoaging and UV damage by acting as the main antioxidant defense against harmful radicals. Additionally, it reduces melanin synthesis by inhibiting tyrosinase, which may benefit patients with hyperpigmentation conditions such as melasma [38, 39]. Furthermore, vitamin C is employed in clinical practice as a potential treatment for various skin conditions, including porphyria cutanea tarda (PCT), herpes zoster (HZ), atopic dermatitis (AD), postherpetic neuralgia (PHN), and malignant melanoma [40].

6.4.1 Potential of Vitamin C in Acne Treatment

Unfortunately, there is insufficient evidence to support the direct use of vitamin C for treating acne. However, Klock et al. [41] investigated the efficacy of Sodium Ascorbyl Phosphate (SAP), a stable precursor of Vitamin C, in treating and preventing acne vulgaris. The pre-clinical experiments demonstrated that SAP exhibited effective antimicrobial action against *P. acnes* and might reduce UVA-induced sebum oxidation. These findings support its potential as an effective therapeutic agent for acne vulgaris. Additionally, Klock and his colleagues conducted a 12-week open-label clinical trial with 60 participants, comparing a 5% SAP lotion to a 5% benzoyl peroxide (BP) cream. The results showed that the SAP lotion had superior efficacy, with 76.9% of participants exhibiting good to excellent improvement in acne symptoms, compared to 60.9% for the BP cream. Notably, SAP did not cause the skin irritation commonly associated with BP, making it a promising alternative to traditional acne treatments [41]. Another *in vitro* study by Lee et al. [29] revealed that magnesium ascorbyl phosphate reduced the expression of antimicrobial peptides, proinflammatory cytokines, matrix metalloproteinases, and Toll-like receptor-4 (TLR-4) in cultured sebocytes, suggesting that it may mitigate the inflammatory responses associated with acne vulgaris [29].

6.4.2 Synergistic Effects of Vitamin C in Acne Treatment Regimens

Recent pre-clinical studies have found a synergistic effect of the combination of Adapalene and Vitamin C that improves overall therapeutic efficacy and cosmetic acceptability. Vitamin C offers protection against UV radiation, which is particularly crucial when using adapalene, a synthetic retinoid that increases skin sensitivity to sunlight. Additionally, Vitamin C has been shown to reduce common side effects of adapalene, such as irritation, dryness, erythema, and peeling, thereby enhancing patient adherence [42, 43]. Interestingly, microneedling with topical vitamin C has demonstrated efficacy in the treatment of atrophic post-acne scars in several clinical studies [44–46].

Administration of oral vitamin C does not raise skin levels beyond plasma saturation; therefore, additional oral dosing is ineffective for those with adequate levels. Nonetheless, topical application has challenges due to vitamin C's instability and susceptibility to oxidation, requiring high-quality formulations to ensure clinical efficacy [39, 47, 48].

6.5 Vitamin E

Vitamin E is one of the fat-soluble vitamins and refers to a class of fat-soluble compounds with unique antioxidant properties. It naturally exists in eight chemical forms: four tocopherol forms (alpha-, beta-, gamma-, and delta-tocopherol) and four tocotrienol forms (alpha-, beta-, gamma-, and delta-tocotrienol) [49]. Among these, alpha-tocopherol is the only form that meets human nutritional requirements, while the others are metabolized and excreted by the liver [50]. Vitamin E is abundant in many foods, including vegetable oils, fruit seeds, whole grains, and nuts; therefore, deficiency is rare and typically results from dietary fat indigestion rather than a lack of vitamin E intake [49, 51, 52].

Vitamin E has long been associated with skin health, mainly due to its antioxidant properties that protect collagen and glycosaminoglycan production from alteration caused by reactive oxygen species (ROS) [53]. It also plays a crucial role in maintaining membrane integrity and may influence the aging process. This is particularly noticeable in cosmetic and skin care products, as many over-the-counter (OTC) anti-aging formulations contain vitamin E [54]. Additionally, topical formulations that combine vitamin E with vitamin C, retinol, and phytonadione have been shown to moderately reduce wrinkles and dark under-eye circles [55]. In the clinical context, studies have indicated that Vitamin E is an effective therapeutic option for treating various dermatological conditions, including yellow nail syndrome, lichen, and macular amyloidosis, subcorneal pustular dermatosis, and granuloma annulare [56–60]. Additionally, various studies found an inverse relationship between serum vitamin E levels and the risk of chronic inflammatory skin conditions, such as psoriasis, atopic dermatitis, vitiligo, and acne vulgaris [61].

6.5.1 Vitamin E in Combination Therapies for Acne Vulgaris

Several studies have revealed that vitamin E levels tend to be lower in patients with acne. El-Akawi et al. [62] demonstrated that plasma vitamin E concentrations were significantly lower in acne patients compared to controls (5.4 vs. 5.9 mg/L, $P = 0.05$) [62]. Additionally, the results showed that patients with severe acne had markedly lower plasma levels of vitamins A and E compared to those with mild acne and age-matched healthy controls. Similarly, a study by Ozuguz et al. [63] involving 94 acne patients reported that levels of vitamin A, zinc, and vitamin E were lower in these patients compared to healthy individuals [63].

Although no clinical studies specifically recommend the use of vitamin E in the treatment of acne vulgaris, a study by Ayres Jr. and Mihan [64] proposed a treatment regimen for 98 patients with acne vulgaris that excluded antibiotics. Instead, the treatment included a combination of vitamins A and E to correct abnormal sebaceous follicular keratinization, thereby inhibiting the formation of milia and comedones, thus preventing *P. acnes* growth environment. Additionally, they found that vitamin E might reduce lipid peroxidation of sebum, which mitigated acne-related inflammation [64]. An RCT involving 168 participants aged 13 to 40 years investigated the efficacy and safety of an oral therapy combining lactoferrin, vitamin E, and zinc for treating mild to moderate acne vulgaris. The treatment group showed a significant reduction in acne lesions, including comedones and inflammatory lesions, with the most pronounced improvement observed at week 10. Sebum levels also notably decreased at week 12. The trial concluded that this combination therapy effectively alleviates mild to moderate acne without any reported side effects. Interestingly, female patients responded more rapidly and favorably to the treatment than male patients [65].

6.5.2 The Role of Vitamin E in Mitigating the Side Effects of Acne Vulgaris Treatments

Vitamin E has been utilized to reduce the adverse effects of isotretinoin at high doses. Nonetheless, recent research showed that vitamin E does not significantly minimize retinoid-related adverse reactions when coupled with isotretinoin for acne treatment [66, 67]. On the other hand, vitamin E can mitigate the adverse effects of benzoyl peroxide (BP) used in acne treatment by reducing the free radicals generated and the depletion of antioxidants caused by BP. *In vitro* studies have demonstrated that in keratinocytes exposed to BP; vitamin E levels drop by 50% within the first 30 min [68]. Moreover, vitamin E can prevent BP-induced lipid peroxidation [69]. These findings suggest that topical vitamin E may reduce BP's adverse effects and restore vitamin E levels in the skin.

While vitamin E is generally considered safe, a systematic review has indicated that daily doses exceeding 150 IU may be associated with increased mortality rates. This risk may be due to inhibition of platelet aggregation, as observed in some *in vitro* studies. Moreover, vitamin E has been shown to interact with medications such as anticoagulants and antiplatelet drugs, potentially enhancing their effects and leading to adverse outcomes [70].

6.6 Vitamin B3

Vitamin B3, commonly known as Niacin, is a water-soluble vitamin that converts into nicotinamide, which serves as a precursor for nicotinamide adenine dinucleotide (NAD), a key molecule essential for ATP synthesis and oxidative phosphorylation reactions in the body. Niacin also acts as a cofactor in over 200 biochemical reactions, emphasizing its importance in various cellular and metabolic processes [71]. Vitamin B3 is widely available in various diets, including animal-based sources such as meat, fish, and poultry, as well as plant-based sources like grains, legumes, and nuts [72].

6.6.1 Rationale for Vitamin D Use in Acne Treatment

Niacinamide, or nicotinamide, is used in the treatment and prevention of various dermatological conditions, including acne vulgaris, psoriasis, wound healing, and skin cancer. It is also employed to prevent and improve skin tone abnormalities [73]. Nicotinamide has demonstrated anti-inflammatory properties by inhibiting mast cell dysregulation and the release of lysosomal enzymes [74]. Additionally, an *in vitro* study also revealed that nicotinamide suppressed IL-8 production induced by *P.acnes* in keratinocytes by modulating the NF-κB and MAPK pathways [75]. It also maintains skin barrier function, promoting microbiota health, and potentially inhibiting *P. acnes* proliferation [74, 77].

6.6.2 Clinical Evidence on Niacinamide Efficacy in Acne Vulgaris Treatment

Several clinical studies have demonstrated the safety and efficacy of niacinamide in the treatment of acne vulgaris, either alone or in combination with other dietary supplements. A Japanese RCT involving 100 healthy women demonstrated that topical 2% niacinamide significantly reduced the sebum excretion rate and casual sebum levels [76]. Furthermore, Kaymak and Onder [78] found that a 4% niacinamide-containing gel was safe and effective in reducing pustules and relieving symptoms in patients with mild to moderate acne [78]. In a split-face RCT conducted by Temper et al. [79], patients applied a ceramide and niacinamide-containing moisturizer (CCM) to one side of the face and a hydrophilic cream to the other. After 2 months, the CCM group showed significant improvement in non-inflammatory, inflammatory, and total acne counts compared to the hydrophilic cream group, suggesting its potential role in enhancing acne lesion healing and reducing skin irritations, thereby optimizing outcomes in mild to moderate acne vulgaris treatment [79]. Various clinical trials have compared topical niacinamide 4% or 5% to clindamycin 1% antibiotic gel for mild to moderate acne vulgaris. However, the results of these studies have been controversial, indicating the need for additional investigations with larger sample sizes and longer durations [80–85].

Furthermore, Nicomide, a formulation combining nicotinamide, copper, zinc, and folic acid, was tested in 198 patients with acne vulgaris and rosacea in a multicenter, open-label trial called Nicomide Improvement in Clinical Outcomes Study (NICOS), assessed the improvement of inflammatory lesions and patient satisfaction at 4 and 8 weeks of treatment. After 4 weeks, 79% of patients reported moderate to marked improvement, which persisted through the 8 weeks. Additionally, Nicomide may serve as an effective alternative to oral antibiotics for treating acne and rosacea, as the study found no significant difference in therapeutic response between patients treated with Nicomide alone and those treated with a combination of Nicomide and oral antibiotics [86]. Similarly, in another 8-week, open-label, prospective multicenter study, 235 patients with inflammatory acne vulgaris were given NicAzel, a novel dietary supplement containing nicotinamide, folic acid, azelaic acid, copper, zinc, and pyridoxine. NicAzel supplementation resulted in significant improvements in acne severity and overall appearance [87].

Nicotinamide is generally considered safe for both oral and topical use, with no reports of major adverse effects. However, some topical side effects, such as itching, burning, and mild dermatitis, have been observed, which are similar to those commonly seen with other topical medications [88, 89]. Nicotinamide presents as a potential, affordable, and safe treatment for acne vulgaris without the risk of antibiotic resistance. Nevertheless, additional evidence from well-designed clinical trials with large population sizes and long follow-up durations is necessary to be recommended as a standard treatment.

6.7 Vitamin B12

Vitamin B12, also known as cobalamin due to its cobalt content, is a water-soluble vitamin that is biologically active in the forms of methylcobalamin and 5-deoxyadenosylcobalamin [90]. Cobalamin plays a crucial role in myelination, central nervous system (CNS) development, and the production of healthy red blood cells [90–92]. Vitamin B12 acts as a cofactor for methionine synthase, facilitating the synthesis of methionine. Methionine is then used to produce S-adenosylmethionine, a compound involved in the methylation of nearly 100 different substrates, including DNA and RNA. Vitamin B12 deficiency is one of the most prevalent vitamin deficiencies, leading to megaloblastic anemia, neurological symptoms, and various psychiatric changes. Additionally, cutaneous manifestations of cobalamin deficiency include hyperpigmentation, changes in hair and nails, and oral alterations such as glossitis [93]. Vitamin B12 is naturally present in various foods, primarily sourced from animals, including red meat, poultry, seafood, eggs, and dairy products [92, 94, 95].

6.7.1 The Link Between Vitamin B12 and Acne Development

Unlike other vitamins, Vitamin B12 has been linked to the development of acne or acne-like eruptions, with a documented positive correlation between elevated serum vitamin B12 levels and acne in case reports as early as 1958 [96–103]. Another case study further supports this link, in which a patient with pernicious anemia who received an intramuscular dose of 5000 μg of hydroxocobalamin reported a significant acne eruption that cleared within 3 months after discontinuing the drug [104]. Furthermore, a cross-sectional study by Kang et al. [105] suggested that skin microbiota and metabolic interactions, particularly involving *P. acnes*, contribute to acne pathogenesis. The study found that vitamin B12 supplementation inhibited the biosynthetic pathway in *P. acnes*, leading to increased porphyrin production levels in in *P. acnes*, which can trigger inflammation linked to acne development [105]. Boreiil et al. [106] further confirmed that high levels of porphyrin production by *P. acnes* induce inflammation and acne pathogenesis, with treatments that reduced porphyrin levels led to clinical improvement, whereas patients with poor outcomes exhibited no reduction in porphyrin levels [106].

6.7.2 Vitamin B12 and Isotretinoin Therapy

Clinical research has connected isotretinoin treatment for acne vulgaris with reduced serum levels of cobalamin, and folic acid, which may lead to neuropsychiatric side effects and occlusive vascular diseases. Therefore, it is recommended that Vitamin B12 and folic acid supplementation be administered under medical supervision before and during isotretinoin therapy [96, 107–110].

6.8 Minerals Overview

Minerals are naturally occurring, inorganic substances that are typically solid. Dietary minerals are categorized into two groups based on the required intake amounts: macrominerals and microminerals. Macrominerals, needed in larger amounts, include calcium, phosphorus, sodium, chloride, sulfur, and potassium. Microminerals, required in smaller quantities, include iron, zinc, selenium, iodine, copper, chromium, fluoride, and manganese. Since almost everything we eat and drink contains minerals, deficiencies are rare, and supplementation is generally unnecessary. Furthermore, Mineral interactions are complex, therefore supplementation requires careful consideration. The existing literature on mineral supplements for treating acne vulgaris is limited, with the notable exception of zinc, although other minerals like sulfur and selenium also have some supporting evidence for their roles.

6.9 Zinc

Zinc is an essential micronutrient that is vital for numerous physiological functions. It plays a multifaceted role in various metabolic processes as an essential cofactor in over 300 metalloenzymes and 2000 transcription factors. It also regulates gene transcription through histone deacetylation and zinc-finger motif-containing proteins. Moreover, zinc is vital for DNA and RNA polymerase function, supporting cell replication, immune activity, and wound repair [111]. It can be obtained from a diverse range of dietary sources, both plant- and animal-based. Animal sources rich in zinc include seafood, eggs, and meat, while plant-based sources include whole grains, beans, and nuts [112].

Certain groups are at a higher risk of zinc deficiency, including patients with gastrointestinal diseases like inflammatory bowel disease (IBD), which includes ulcerative colitis and Crohn's disease, as well as patients with malnutrition, malabsorption syndromes, and alcoholism [113–115]. Vegetarians are also at risk, as plant-based foods generally contain lower levels of zinc compared to animal-based sources [116]. During pregnancy, zinc requirements increase to support fetal growth, with a recommended intake of 3 mg/day more than that of non-pregnant women in the same age group; this requirement further increases by 4 mg/day during breastfeeding [117, 118].

Zinc supplementation effectively prevents upper respiratory infections and diarrhea, particularly in malnourished children. Additionally, zinc can delay the progression of age-related macular degeneration when combined with antioxidants and has demonstrated effectiveness in treating Wilson disease [115]. Zinc is beneficial in treating various dermatological conditions, including neoplasms like basal cell carcinoma, inflammatory conditions such as hidradenitis suppurativa and acne rosacea, hair loss issues, and pigmentation disorders like melasma [119, 120].

6.9.1 Rationale for Zinc Use in Acne Vulgaris Treatment

The association between zinc deficiency and acne vulgaris was first recognized in the 1970s by Fitzherbert [121], who observed improved acne symptoms in patients with acrodermatitis enteropathica following zinc supplementation. Later research by Michaëlsson [122] further confirmed this observation, revealing that individuals with acne had significantly lower zinc levels compared to others. Due to its anti-inflammatory properties, zinc is effective in treating acne by inhibiting inflammatory mediators such as nitric oxide, TNF-α, and IL-6, as well as toll-like receptors expressed by keratinocytes [111, 123]. Additionally, zinc directly inhibits the proliferation of *P. acnes* and suppresses sebaceous gland activity by reducing the synthesis of dihydrotestosterone (DHT), which activates sebaceous gland function [63, 124, 125].

6.9.2 Clinical Evidence on Zinc Efficacy in Acne Vulgaris Treatment

A systematic review by Yee et al. [126], involving 25 studies with 2445 participants, found that acne patients had lower zinc levels compared to controls. Additionally, significant improvements in acne were observed when zinc was administered, either orally or topically, compared to placebo or active treatments like clindamycin with benzoyl peroxide or topical tea tree extract [126]. Furthermore, a study by Tino et al. [127] involving 100 patients with mild to moderate acne demonstrated a significant reduction in Global Acne Grading System (GAGS) scores in both the zinc sulfate and lymecycline antibiotic groups. However, there was no statistically significant difference in GAGS score reduction between the two groups. Notably, the zinc sulfate group showed greater improvements in the Acne Quality of Life Assessment (AQoL) compared to the lymecycline group [127]. Similarly, a study by Eman Salah [128] involving 60 patients with moderate to severe acne compared two groups: one receiving zinc and low-dose isotretinoin, and the control group receiving the standard dose of isotretinoin. The results showed no significant difference in efficacy between the two groups. Additionally, 76.7% of participants in the control group experienced treatment-related side effects, compared to only 20% in the experimental group. Thus, adding zinc to isotretinoin not only achieved comparable results to the standard dose of isotretinoin but also reduced side effects and treatment costs [128].

6.9.3 Drug Interactions and Zinc Supplementation

Drug interactions are crucial to consider when supplementing zinc. For instance, zinc decreases the absorption of quinolone, tetracycline antibiotics, and penicillamine, so a 2-h gap between doses is recommended [129, 130]. Moreover, hydrochlorothiazide treatment can increase zinc excretion by up to 60%, potentially requiring long-term supplementation [131]. Iron supplements can also lower zinc levels, and zinc supplements can cause copper deficiency, leading to sideroblastic anemia [132–134].

6.10 Sulfur

Sulfur is known for its keratolytic, bacteriostatic, and antifungal properties, which have been used in acne treatment for decades. It is converted to hydrogen sulfide in keratinocytes, which may have the ability to degrade keratin [135]. In 1966, a Canadian study by Wilkinson et al. evaluated the efficacy of a topical cream containing 10% benzoyl peroxide and 2–5% sulfur in treating various forms of acne, including comedonic, papular, pustular, and cystic acne, in 113 patients. The treatment produced "good" to "excellent" results with minimal side effects, establishing it as a standard regimen in clinical practice [136]. Moreover, a study by Hashem et al. [137] demonstrated that sulfur nanoparticle formulations (SNPs) exhibit a potent antibacterial effect against multi-drug-resistant strains of *Staphylococcus aureus* (*S. aureus*) and *Staphylococcus epidermidis* (*S. epidermidis*) isolated from acne lesions. Besides treating acne vulgaris, sulfur is also effective in managing dandruff, scabies, and various other skin conditions [138].

6.11 Selenium

Selenium is an essential trace mineral with significant roles in thyroid function, reproduction, DNA synthesis, and protection from oxidative stress, inflammation, and infection [139–142]. A systematic review and meta-analysis by Lv et al. [143], which included 27 studies involving 1315 patients and 7181 healthy controls, revealed that low selenium levels are associated with atopic dermatitis, acne vulgaris, chloracne, and psoriasis. This finding suggests that selenium deficiency might be linked to multiple skin disorders [143]. Selenium's antioxidant and anti-inflammatory actions, combined with its role in sebum regulation, have made it a valuable component in the treatment regimens of acne vulgaris, particularly when used alongside zinc and vitamin E. This combination has been shown to reduce malondialdehyde levels, IL-8, and the count of inflammatory lesions [144]. In 1990, Michaëlsson measured selenium levels in whole blood and plasma among young adults with inflammatory acne and compared them to healthy controls. The results revealed a reduction in selenium levels in both whole blood and plasma in male and female acne patients compared to the controls [145]. More recently, a case-control study found that patients with acne vulgaris had significantly lower serum levels of zinc, selenium, and vitamin D compared to controls, with the lowest levels in those with more severe acne [146]. Therefore, elevated selenium levels may act as a protective factor and exhibit potential therapeutic benefits as an adjuvant therapy in the treatment of acne vulgaris; however, further research is necessary to confirm its effectiveness.

References

1. Carazo A, Macáková K, Matoušová K, Krčmová LK, Protti M, Mladěnka P. Vitamin A update: forms, sources, kinetics, detection, function, deficiency, therapeutic use and toxicity. Nutrients. 2021;13(5):1703.
2. D'Ambrosio DN, Clugston RD, Blaner WS. Vitamin A metabolism: an update. Nutrients. 2011;3(1):63–103.
3. Dreno B, Kang S, Leyden J, York J. Update: mechanisms of topical retinoids in acne. J Drugs Dermatol. 2022;21(7):734–40.
4. Draghici C, Miulescu R, Petca R, Petca A, Dumitraşcu MC, Şandru F. Teratogenic effect of isotretinoin in both fertile females and males (Review). Exp Ther Med. 2021;21(5):534. https://doi.org/10.3892/etm.2021.9966.
5. Layton A. The use of isotretinoin in acne. Dermatoendocrinol. 2009;1(3):162–9.
6. US Food and Drug Administration. iPLEDGE risk evaluation and mitigation strategy (REMS) [Internet]. 2023. Available at: https://www.fda.gov/drugs/postmarket-drug-safety-information-patients-and-providers/ipledge-risk-evaluation-and-mitigation-strategy-rems. Accessed 02 Mar 2025.
7. Sadeghzadeh-Bazargan A, Ghassemi M, Goodarzi A, Roohaninasab M, Najar Nobari N, Behrangi E. Systematic review of low-dose isotretinoin for treatment of acne vulgaris: Focus on indication, dosage, regimen, efficacy, safety, satisfaction, and follow up, based on clinical studies. Dermatol Ther. 2021;34(1):e14438.
8. Antonucci R, Locci C, Clemente MG, Chicconi E, Antonucci L. Vitamin D deficiency in childhood: old lessons and current challenges. J Pediatr Endocrinol Metab. 2018;31(3):247–60.
9. Chang S-W, Lee H-C. Vitamin D and health—the missing vitamin in humans. Pediatr Neonatol. 2019;60(3):237–44.
10. Mostafa WZ, Hegazy RA. Vitamin D and the skin: Focus on a complex relationship: a review. J Adv Res. 2015;6(6):793–804.
11. Arnson Y, Amital H, Shoenfeld Y. Vitamin D and autoimmunity: new aetiological and therapeutic considerations. Ann Rheum Dis. 2007;66(9):1137–42.

12. Ahmed Mohamed A, Salah Ahmed EM, Abdel-Aziz RTA, Eldeeb Abdallah HH, El-Hanafi H, Hussein G, et al. The impact of active vitamin D administration on the clinical outcomes of acne vulgaris. J Dermatolog Treat. 2021;32(7):756–61.
13. AlGhamdi K, Kumar A, Moussa N. The role of vitamin D in melanogenesis with an emphasis on vitiligo. Indian J Dermatol Venereol Leprol. 2013;79(6):750–8.
14. Lin X, Meng X, Song Z. Vitamin D and alopecia areata: possible roles in pathogenesis and potential implications for therapy. Am J Transl Res. 2019;11(9):5285–300.
15. Reichrath J, Schuler CH, Seifert M, Zouboulis CH, Tilgen W. The vitamin D endocrine system of human sebocytes. Exp Dermatol. 2006;15(8):643–8.
16. Agak GW, Qin M, Nobe J, Kim M-H, Krutzik SR, Tristan GR, et al. Propionibacterium acnes induces an IL-17 response in acne vulgaris that is regulated by vitamin A and vitamin D. J Invest Dermatol. 2014;134(2):366–73.
17. Alhetheli G, Elneam AIA, Alsenaid A. Vitamin D levels in patients with and without acne and its relation to acne severity: a case-control study. Clin Cosmet Investig Dermatol. 2020;13:759–65.
18. Lee WJ, Choi YH, Sohn MY, Lee S-J, Kim DW. Expression of inflammatory biomarkers from cultured sebocytes was influenced by treatment with vitamin D. Indian J Dermatol. 2013;58(4):327.
19. Schauber J, Dorschner RA, Coda AB, Büchau AS, Liu PT, Kiken D, et al. Injury enhances TLR2 function and antimicrobial peptide expression through a vitamin D-dependent mechanism. J Clin Invest. 2007;117(3):803–11.
20. Yildizgören MT, Togral AK. Preliminary evidence for vitamin D deficiency in nodulocystic acne. Dermatoendocrinol. 2014;6(1):e983687.
21. Stewart TJ, Bazergy C. Hormonal and dietary factors in acne vulgaris versus controls. Dermatoendocrinol. 2018;10(1):e1442160.
22. Lim S-K, Ha J-M, Lee Y-H, Lee Y, Seo Y-J, Kim C-D, et al. Comparison of vitamin D levels in patients with and without acne: a case-control study combined with a randomized controlled trial. PLoS One. 2016;11(8):e0161162.
23. Al-Taiar A, AlKhabbaz M, Rahman A, Al-Sabah R, Shaban L, Akhtar S. Plasma 25-hydroxy vitamin D is not associated with acne vulgaris. Nutrients. 2018;10(10):1525.
24. Toossi P, Azizian Z, Yavari H, Fakhim TH, Amini SHS, Enamzade R. Serum 25-hydroxy vitamin D levels in patients with acne vulgaris and its association with disease severity. Clin Cases Miner Bone Metab. 2015;12(3):238–42.
25. Wang M, Zhou Y, Yan Y. Vitamin D status and efficacy of vitamin D supplementation in acne patients: A systematic review and meta-analysis. J Cosmet Dermatol. 2021;20(12):3802–7. https://doi.org/10.1111/jocd.14057. Epub 2021 Apr 15. PMID: 33690970. URL: https://onlinelibrary.wiley.com/doi/10.1111/jocd.14057.
26. Abdel Wahab HM, Ali AK, Ragaie MH. Calcipotriol: A novel tool in treatment of acne vulgaris. Dermatol Ther. 2022;35(9):e15690.
27. Amarnath SS, Kumar V, Barik S. Vitamin D and calcium and bioavailability of calcium in various calcium salts. Indian J Orthop. 2023;57(Suppl 1):62–9.
28. Li Y, Schellhorn HE. New developments and novel therapeutic perspectives for vitamin C. J Nutr. 2007;137(10):2171–84.
29. Lee WJ, Kim SL, Choe YS, Jang YH, Lee S-J, Kim DW. Magnesium ascorbyl phosphate regulates the expression of inflammatory biomarkers in cultured sebocytes. Ann Dermatol. 2015;27(4):376.
30. Lykkesfeldt J, Michels AJ, Frei B. Vitamin C. Adv Nutr. 2014;5(1):16–8.
31. Olmedo JM, Yiannias JA, Windgassen EB, Gornet MK. Scurvy: a disease almost forgotten. Int J Dermatol. 2006;45(8):909–13.
32. Hirschmann JV, Raugi GJ. Adult scurvy. J Am Acad Dermatol. 1999;41(6):895–906; quiz 907.
33. Carr AC, Frei B. Toward a new recommended dietary allowance for vitamin C based on antioxidant and health effects in humans. Am J Clin Nutr. 1999;69(6):1086–107.

34. Frei B, England L, Ames BN. Ascorbate is an outstanding antioxidant in human blood plasma. Proc Natl Acad Sci USA. 1989;86(16):6377–81.
35. Taddei S, Virdis A, Ghiadoni L, Magagna A, Salvetti A. Vitamin C improves endothelium-dependent vasodilation by restoring nitric oxide activity in essential hypertension. Circulation. 1998;97(22):2222–9.
36. Gershoff SN. Vitamin C (ascorbic acid): new roles, new requirements? Nutr Rev. 1993;51(11):313–26.
37. Jacob RA, Sotoudeh G. Vitamin C function and status in chronic disease. Nutr Clin Care. 2002;5(2):66–74.
38. Correia G, Magina S. Efficacy of topical vitamin C in melasma and photoaging: a systematic review. J Cosmet Dermatol. 2023;22(7):1938–45.
39. Pullar JM, Carr AC, Vissers MCM. The roles of vitamin C in skin health. Nutrients. 2017;9(8):866.
40. Wang K, Jiang H, Li W, Qiang M, Dong T, Li H. Role of vitamin C in skin diseases. Front Physiol. 2018;9:819.
41. Klock J, Ikeno H, Ohmori K, Nishikawa T, Vollhardt J, Schehlmann V. Sodium ascorbyl phosphate shows in vitro and in vivo efficacy in the prevention and treatment of acne vulgaris. Int J Cosmet Sci. 2005;27(3):171–6.
42. Vasanth S, Dubey A, Ravi GS, Lewis SA, Ghate VM, El-Zahaby SA, et al. Development and investigation of vitamin C-enriched adapalene-loaded transfersome gel: a collegial approach for the treatment of acne vulgaris. AAPS PharmSciTech. 2020;21(2):61.
43. Jain A, Garg NK, Jain A, Kesharwani P, Jain AK, Nirbhavane P, et al. A synergistic approach of adapalene-loaded nanostructured lipid carriers, and vitamin C co-administration for treating acne. Drug Dev Ind Pharm. 2016;42(6):897–905.
44. Abbas MAM, Elgamal EEAE, Zaky MS, Elsaie ML. Microneedling with topical vitamin C versus microneedling with topical insulin in the treatment of atrophic post-acne scars: a split-face study. Dermatol Ther. 2022;35(5):e15376.
45. Mohhmed R, Abo EM. Efficacy of diamond microdermabrasion with topical vitamin C in treatment of acne scars. Sohag Medical Journal. 2019;23(1):207–12.
46. Chawla S. Split face comparative study of microneedling with PRP versus microneedling with vitamin C in treating atrophic post acne scars. J Cutan Aesthet Surg. 2014;7(4):209–12.
47. Levine M, Rumsey SC, Daruwala R, Park JB, Wang Y. Criteria and recommendations for vitamin C intake. JAMA. 1999;281(15):1415–23.
48. Al-Niaimi F, Chiang NYZ. Topical vitamin C and the skin: mechanisms of action and clinical applications. J Clin Aesthet Dermatol. 2017;10(7):14–7.
49. Modern nutrition in health and disease. Diabetes. 1956;5(6):496–6.
50. Traber MG. Vitamin E regulatory mechanisms. Annu Rev Nutr. 2007;27:347–62.
51. Shahidi F, Pinaffi-Langley ACC, Fuentes J, Speisky H, de Camargo AC. Vitamin E as an essential micronutrient for human health: common, novel, and unexplored dietary sources. Free Radic Biol Med. 2021;176:312–21.
52. Bunnell RH, Keating J, Quaresimo A, Parman GK. Alpha-tocopherol content of foods. Am J Clin Nutr. 1965;17(1):1–10.
53. Tanaka H, Okada T, Konishi H, Tsuji T. The effect of reactive oxygen species on the biosynthesis of collagen and glycosaminoglycans in cultured human dermal fibroblasts. Arch Dermatol Res. 1993;285(6):352–5.
54. Ochi H, Takeda S. The two sides of vitamin E supplementation. Gerontology. 2015;61(4):319–26.
55. Mitsuishi T, Shimoda T, Mitsui Y, Kuriyama Y, Kawana S. The effects of topical application of phytonadione, retinol and vitamins C and E on infraorbital dark circles and wrinkles of the lower eyelids. J Cosmet Dermatol. 2004;3(2):73–5.
56. Ashamalla L, Maurice M, Sidhom K. Topical vitamin E in granuloma annulare. Int J Dermatol. 1988;27(5):348.
57. Terao M, Nishida K, Murota H, Katayama I. Clinical effect of tocoretinate on lichen and macular amyloidosis. J Dermatol. 2011;38(2):179–84.

58. Ayres S, Mihan R. Letter: subcorneal pustular dermatosis controlled by vitamin E. Arch Dermatol. 1974;109(6):914.
59. Al Hawsawi K, Pope E. Yellow nail syndrome. Pediatr Dermatol. 2010;27(6):675–6.
60. Norton L. Further observations on the yellow nail syndrome with therapeutic effects of oral alpha-tocopherol. Cutis. 1985;36(6):457–62.
61. Liu X, Yang G, Luo M, Lan Q, Shi X, Deng H, et al. Serum vitamin E levels and chronic inflammatory skin diseases: a systematic review and meta-analysis. PLoS One. 2021;16(12):e0261259.
62. El-Akawi Z, Abdel-Latif N, Abdul-Razzak K. Does the plasma level of vitamins A and E affect acne condition? Clin Exp Dermatol. 2006;31(3):430–4.
63. Ozuguz P, Dogruk Kacar S, Ekiz O, Takci Z, Balta I, Kalkan G. Evaluation of serum vitamins A and E and zinc levels according to the severity of acne vulgaris. Cutan Ocul Toxicol. 2014;33(2):99–102.
64. Ayres S Jr, Mihan R. Acne vulgaris: therapy directed at pathophysiologic defects. Cutis. 1981;28:41–2.
65. Sukwa TY, Mulenga M, Chisdaka N, Roskell NS, Scott TR. A randomized, double-blind, placebo-controlled field trial to determine the efficacy and safety of Malarone (atovaquone/proguanil) for the prophylaxis of malaria in Zambia. Am J Trop Med Hyg. 1999;60(4):521–5.
66. Strauss JS, Gottlieb AB, Jones T, Koo JY, Leyden JJ, Lucky A, et al. Concomitant administration of vitamin E does not change the side effects of isotretinoin as used in acne vulgaris: a randomized trial. J Am Acad Dermatol. 2000;43(5 Pt 1):777–84.
67. Kus S, Gün D, Demirçay Z, Sur H. Vitamin E does not reduce the side-effects of isotretinoin in the treatment of acne vulgaris. Int J Dermatol. 2005;44(3):248–51.
68. Valacchi G, Rimbach G, Saliou C, Weber SU, Packer L. Effect of benzoyl peroxide on antioxidant status, NF-κB activity and interleukin-1α gene expression in human keratinocytes. Toxicology. 2001;165(2–3):225–34.
69. Rota C, Tomasi A, Iannone A. Alpha-tocopherol amplifies benzoyl peroxide free radical decomposition in a chemical system. Free Radic Res. 2006;40(6):637–45.
70. Miller ER, Pastor-Barriuso R, Dalal D, Riemersma RA, Appel LJ, Guallar E. Meta-analysis: high-dosage vitamin E supplementation may increase all-cause mortality. Ann Intern Med. 2005;142(1):37–46.
71. Karthikeyan K, Thappa DM. Pellagra and skin. Int J Dermatol. 2002;41(8):476–81.
72. Çatak J. Determination of niacin profiles in some animal and plant based foods by high performance liquid chromatography: association with healthy nutrition. J Anim Sci Technol. 2019;61(3):138–46.
73. Boo YC. Mechanistic basis and clinical evidence for the applications of nicotinamide (niacinamide) to control skin aging and pigmentation. Antioxidants (Basel). 2021;10(8):1315.
74. Wohlrab J, Kreft D. Niacinamide—mechanisms of action and its topical use in dermatology. Skin Pharmacol Physiol. 2014;27(6):311–5.
75. Grange PA, Raingeaud J, Calvez V, Dupin N. Nicotinamide inhibits propionibacterium acnes-induced IL-8 production in keratinocytes through the NF-kappaB and MAPK pathways. J Dermatol Sci. 2009;56(2):106–12.
76. Draelos ZD, Matsubara A, Smiles K. The effect of 2% niacinamide on facial sebum production. J Cosmet Laser Ther. 2006;8(2):96–101.
77. Fivenson DP. The mechanisms of action of nicotinamide and zinc in inflammatory skin disease. Cutis. 2006;77(1 Suppl):5–10.
78. Kaymak Y, Onder M. An investigation of efficacy of topical niacinamide for the treatment of mild and moderate acne vulgaris. J Turk Acad Dermatol. 2008;2(4):jtad82402a.
79. Tempark T, Shem A, Lueangarun S. Efficacy of ceramides and niacinamide-containing moisturizer versus hydrophilic cream in combination with topical anti-acne treatment in mild to moderate acne vulgaris: A split face, double-blinded, randomized controlled trial. J Cosmet Dermatol. 2024;23(5):1758–65.

80. Shahmoradi Z, Iraji F, Siadat AH, Ghorbaini A. Comparison of topical 5% nicotinamid gel versus 2% clindamycin gel in the treatment of the mild-moderate acne vulgaris: a double-blinded randomized clinical trial. J Res Med Sci. 2013;18(2):115–7.
81. Khodaeiani E, Fouladi RF, Amirnia M, Saeidi M, Karimi ER. Topical 4% nicotinamide vs. 1% clindamycin in moderate inflammatory acne vulgaris. Int J Dermatol. 2013;52(8):999–1004.
82. Sardesai VR, Kambli VM. Comparison of efficacy of topical clindamycin and nicotinamide combination with plain clindamycin for the treatment of acne vulgaris and acne resistant to topical antibiotics. Indian J Dermatol Venereol Leprol. 2003;69(2):138–9.
83. Dos SK, Barbhuiya JN, Jana S, Dey SK. Comparative evaluation of clindamycin phosphate 1% and clindamycin phosphate 1% with nicotinamide gel 4% in the treatment of acne vulgaris. Indian J Dermatol Venereol Leprol. 2003;69(1):8–9.
84. Shalita AR, Smith JG, Parish LC, Sofman MS, Chalker DK. Topical nicotinamide compared with clindamycin gel in the treatment of inflammatory acne vulgaris. Int J Dermatol. 1995;34(6):434–7.
85. Morganti P, Berardesca E, Guarneri B, Guarneri F, Fabrizi G, Palombo P, et al. Topical clindamycin 1% vs. linoleic acid-rich phosphatidylcholine and nicotinamide 4% in the treatment of acne: a multicentre-randomized trial. Int J Cosmet Sci. 2011;33(5):467–76.
86. Niren NM, Torok HM. The nicomide improvement in clinical outcomes study (NICOS): results of an 8-week trial. Cutis. 2006;77(1 Suppl):17–28.
87. Shalita AR, Falcon R, Olansky A, Iannotta P, Akhavan A, Day D, et al. Inflammatory acne management with a novel prescription dietary supplement. J Drugs Dermatol. 2012;11(12):1428–33.
88. Walocko FM, Eber AE, Keri JE, Al-Harbi MA, Nouri K. The role of nicotinamide in acne treatment. Dermatol Ther. 2017;30(5):e12481. https://doi.org/10.1111/dth.12481.
89. Rolfe HM. A review of nicotinamide: treatment of skin diseases and potential side effects. J Cosmet Dermatol. 2014;13(4):324–8.
90. Institute of Medicine (US) Standing Committee on the Scientific Evaluation of Dietary Reference Intakes and its Panel on Folate, Other B Vitamins, and Choline. Dietary reference intakes for thiamin, riboflavin, niacin, vitamin B6, folate, vitamin B12, pantothenic acid, biotin, and choline. Washington, DC: National Academies Press (US); 1998.
91. Allen LH. Vitamin B-12. Adv Nutr. 2012;3(1):54–5.
92. Stabler SP. Vitamin B12. In: Present knowledge in nutrition. Elsevier; 2020. p. 257–71.
93. Brescoll J, Daveluy S. A review of vitamin B12 in dermatology. Am J Clin Dermatol. 2015;16(1):27–33.
94. Watanabe F, Bito T. Vitamin B12 sources and microbial interaction. Exp Biol Med (Maywood). 2018;243(2):148–58.
95. Gille D, Schmid A. Vitamin B12 in meat and dairy products. Nutr Rev. 2015;73(2):106–15.
96. Karadag AS, Tutal E, Ertugrul DT, Akin KO. Effect of isotretinoin treatment on plasma holotranscobalamin, vitamin B12, folic acid, and homocysteine levels: non-controlled study. Int J Dermatol. 2011;50(12):1564–9.
97. Goldblatt S. Vitamin B-12 levels in blood serum in acne-like skin diseases. Hautarzt. 1966;17(3):106–8.
98. Sherertz EF. Acneiform eruption due to "megadose" vitamins B6 and B12. Cutis. 1991;48(2):119–20.
99. Balta I, Ozuguz P. Vitamin B12-induced acneiform eruption. Cutan Ocul Toxicol. 2014;33(2):94–5.
100. Dupré A, Albarel N, Bonafe JL, Christol B, Lassere J. Vitamin B-12 induced acnes. Cutis. 1979;24(2):210–1.
101. Braun-Falco O, Lincke H. The problem of vitamin B6/B12 acne. A contribution on acne medicamentosa (author's transl). MMW Munch Med Wochenschr. 1976;118(6):155–60.
102. Puissant A, Vanbremeersch F, Monfort J. A new iatrogenic dermatosis: acne caused by vitamin B 12. Bull Soc Fr Dermatol Syphiligr. 1967;74(6):813–5.
103. Franceschetti A, Jadassohn W, Paillard R, Hofer R, Golay M. II. démonstrations—demonstrationen. Dermatology (Basel). 1958;116(4–5):331–4.

104. Bahbouhi I, Aboudourib M, Hocar O, Amal S. Vitamin B12 induced acneiform eruption. Heliyon. 2023;9(5):e16120.
105. Kang D, Shi B, Erfe MC, Craft N, Li H. Vitamin B12 modulates the transcriptome of the skin microbiota in acne pathogenesis. Sci Transl Med. 2015;7(293):293ra103.
106. Borelli C, Merk K, Schaller M, Jacob K, Vogeser M, Weindl G, et al. In vivo porphyrin production by P. acnes in untreated acne patients and its modulation by acne treatment. Acta Derm Venereol. 2006;86(4):316–9.
107. Kim HJ, Lee SM, Lee JS, Lee SY, Chung EH, Cho MK, et al. Homocysteine, folic acid, and vitamin B12 levels in patients on isotretinoin therapy for acne vulgaris: a meta-analysis. J Cosmet Dermatol. 2020;19(3):736–45.
108. Mohammed MI, Mahmoud MM, Mikhael W, Abd El Khalik GM. Assessment of serum vitamin B12 level in patients with acne after isotretenoin therapy and its correlation to adverse mood changes. Benha J Appl Sci. 2022;7(4):107–11.
109. Kamal M, Polat M. Effect of different doses of isotretinoin treatment on the levels of serum homocysteine, vitamin B 12 and folic acid in patients with acne vulgaris: a prospective controlled study. J Pak Med Assoc. 2015;65(9):950–3.
110. Gökalp H, Bulur I, Gürer M. Decreased vitamin B12 and folic Acid concentrations in acne patients after isotretinoin therapy: a controlled study. Indian J Dermatol. 2014;59(6):630.
111. Cervantes J, Eber AE, Perper M, Nascimento VM, Nouri K, Keri JE. The role of zinc in the treatment of acne: a review of the literature. Dermatol Ther. 2018;31(1):e12576.
112. Kalita DJ, Pradeepika C. Zinc-containing vegetables, fruits and other food products. In: Zinc: early development, applications, and emerging trends. Boca Raton: CRC Press; 2024. p. 39–48.
113. Ehrlich S, Mark AG, Rinawi F, Shamir R, Assa A. Micronutrient deficiencies in children with inflammatory bowel diseases. Nutr Clin Pract. 2020;35(2):315–22.
114. Siva S, Rubin DT, Gulotta G, Wroblewski K, Pekow J. Zinc deficiency is associated with poor clinical outcomes in patients with inflammatory bowel disease. Inflamm Bowel Dis. 2017;23(1):152–7.
115. Saper RB, Rash R. Zinc: an essential micronutrient. Am Fam Physician. 2009;79(9):768–72.
116. Foster M, Chu A, Petocz P, Samman S. Effect of vegetarian diets on zinc status: a systematic review and meta-analysis of studies in humans. J Sci Food Agric. 2013;93(10):2362–71.
117. Ryu MS, Aydemir ATB. Zinc. In: Marriott BP, Birt DF, Stallings VA, Yates AA, editors. Present knowledge in nutrition. Elsevier; 2020.
118. Institute of Medicine (US) Panel on Micronutrients. Dietary reference intakes for vitamin A, vitamin K, arsenic, boron, chromium, copper, iodine, iron, manganese, molybdenum, nickel, silicon, vanadium, and zinc. Washington, DC: National Academies Press (US); 2001.
119. Gupta M, Mahajan VK, Mehta KS, Chauhan PS. Zinc therapy in dermatology: a review. Dermatol Res Pract. 2014;2014:709152.
120. Searle T, Ali FR, Al-Niaimi F. Zinc in dermatology. J Dermatolog Treat. 2022;33(5):2455–8.
121. Fitzherbert JC. Acne vulgaris-zinc deficiency? Med J Aust. 1976;1(22):848.
122. Michaëlsson G, Vahlquist A, Juhlin L. Serum zinc and retinol-binding protein in acne. Br J Dermatol. 1977;96(3):283–6.
123. Sardana K, Chugh S, Garg VK. The role of zinc in acne and prevention of resistance: have we missed the "base" effect? Int J Dermatol. 2014;53(1):125–7.
124. Sugimoto Y, López-Solache I, Labrie F, Luu-The V. Cations inhibit specifically type I 5α-reductase found in human skin. J Invest Dermatol. 1995;104(5):775–8.
125. Azzouni F, Godoy A, Li Y, Mohler J. The 5 alpha-reductase isozyme family: a review of basic biology and their role in human diseases. Adv Urol. 2012;2012:530121.
126. Yee BE, Richards P, Sui JY, Marsch AF. Serum zinc levels and efficacy of zinc treatment in acne vulgaris: a systematic review and meta-analysis. Dermatol Ther. 2020;33(6):e14252.
127. Tolino E, Skroza N, Mambrin A, Proietti I, Bernardini N, Balduzzi V, et al. An open-label study comparing oral zinc to lymecycline in the treatment of acne vulgaris. J Clin Aesthet Dermatol. 2021;14(5):56–8.

128. Salah E. Oral zinc as a novel adjuvant and sparing therapy for systemic isotretinoin in acne vulgaris: a preliminary comparative study. J Clin Aesthet Dermatol. 2022;15(10):58–61.
129. Lomaestro BM, Bailie GR. Absorption interactions with fluoroquinolones. 1995 update. Drug Saf. 1995;12(5):314–33.
130. Penttilä O, Hurme H, Neuvonen PJ. Effect of zinc sulphate on the absorption of tetracycline and doxycycline in man. Eur J Clin Pharmacol. 1975;9(2–3):131–4.
131. Wester PO. Urinary zinc excretion during treatment with different diuretics. Acta Med Scand. 1980;208(3):209–12.
132. Broun ER, Greist A, Tricot G, Hoffman R, Excessive zinc ingestion. A reversible cause of sideroblastic anemia and bone marrow depression. JAMA. 1990;264(11):1441–3.
133. Willis MS, Monaghan SA, Miller ML, McKenna RW, Perkins WD, Levinson BS, et al. Zinc-induced copper deficiency: a report of three cases initially recognized on bone marrow examination. Am J Clin Pathol. 2005;123(1):125–31.
134. Whittaker P. Iron and zinc interactions in humans. Am J Clin Nutr. 1998;68(2 Suppl):442S–6S.
135. Akhavan A, Bershad S. Topical acne drugs: review of clinical properties, systemic exposure, and safety. Am J Clin Dermatol. 2003;4(7):473–92.
136. Wilkinson RD, Adam JE, Murray JJ, Craig GE. Benzoyl peroxide and sulfur: foundation for acne management. Can Med Assoc J. 1966;95(1):28–9.
137. Hashem NM, Hosny AE-DMS, Abdelrahman AA, Zakeer S. Antimicrobial activities encountered by sulfur nanoparticles combating Staphylococcal species harboring sccmecA recovered from acne vulgaris. AIMS Microbiol. 2021;7(4):481–98.
138. Lin AN, Reimer RJ, Carter DM. Sulfur revisited. J Am Acad Dermatol. 1988;18(3):553–8.
139. Pincemail J, Meziane S. On the potential role of the antioxidant couple vitamin e/selenium taken by the oral route in skin and hair health. Antioxidants (Basel). 2022;11(11):2270.
140. Rayman MP. The importance of selenium to human health. Lancet. 2000;356(9225):233–41.
141. Rayman MP. Selenium and human health. Lancet. 2012;379(9822):1256–68.
142. Hong LK, Diamond AM. Selenium. In: Present knowledge in nutrition. Elsevier; 2020. p. 443–56.
143. Lv J, Ai P, Lei S, Zhou F, Chen S, Zhang Y. Selenium levels and skin diseases: systematic review and meta-analysis. J Trace Elem Med Biol. 2020;62:126548.
144. Podgórska A, Puścion-Jakubik A, Markiewicz-Żukowska R, Gromkowska-Kępka KJ, Socha K. Acne vulgaris and intake of selected dietary nutrients—a summary of information. Healthcare (Basel). 2021;9(6):668.
145. Michaëlsson G. Decreased concentration of selenium in whole blood and plasma in acne vulgaris. Acta Derm Venereol. 1990;70(1):92.
146. Kazeminejad A, Hajheydari Z, Taghian SS, Gholizadeh N. Serum zinc, selenium, and vitamin D levels in patients with acne vulgaris: a case–control study. J Cosmet Dermatol. 2024;23(12):4249–54.

Skin-Gut Axis

7

Esraa M. AlEdani and Aya Mohammed Sharkawy

Contents

7.1 Introduction

Skin and gut -which are the largest organs in the body- have many similar features, both are richly innervated, densely vascularized, complex endocrinal, and highly immunological organs [1].

They are exposed to the external environment and colonized with the large number of microbiota -both commensal and pathogenic-hence it is essential to maintain homeostasis and survival by communicating with each other in a bidirectional manner [2].

E. M. AlEdani (✉)
Basra Medical College, Basrah, Iraq

A. M. Sharkawy
Faculty of Medicine, South Valley University, Qena, Egypt

E. M. AlEdani, H. I. Maibach (eds.), *Nutrition and Acne Vulgaris*, Updates in Clinical Dermatology, https://doi.org/10.1007/978-3-031-83677-0_7

The skin gut axis is a term used for the complicated interaction between the skin and the gut, it is an inseparable, bidirectional communication system between the gut and the skin involving various immune, neural, and endocrine pathways, any microbial imbalance or disruption of the gut integrity may have a significant impact in the skin homeostasis as it plays a crucial role in maintaining overall health and homeostasis [3].

7.2 Mechanism of Interaction

To the best of our knowledge, there are four mechanisms of interaction,

7.2.1 Metabolic Interaction

While The gut is the main organ of metabolism, the skin also is a major metabolic organ. It plays a vital role in vitamin D synthesis [4]. it has a wide range of enzymatic activities that may exceed that of our gut and liver [5].

7.2.2 Nervous System Interaction

Many examples exist of the GI-CNS-skin axis, the most important one is 'zones of referred pain' (Head's zones), i.e. the projection of pain into defined skin regions induced by pathological changes in visceral organs [6].

Recently the studies reported some Molecules synthesized by gut bacteria with the potential to modify skin either directly or indirectly.

For example:

- Short-chain fatty acids, e.g. butyrate, acetate, and propionate may have Anti-inflammatory effects.
- Tryptamine leads to Itching.
- Trimethylamine has a vital role in Prevention of keratinocyte fragility.
- Acetylcholine plays a role in Barrier function.
- GABA has a possible effect on the Inhibition of itching.
- Dopamine has a role in Inhibition of hair growth.
- Serotonin plays a role in Melatonin synthesis [1].
- Endocrinal interaction

It is integral to the GI-CNS-skin axis, it is a neuroendocrinal circuit, after ingesting nutrients, gut endocrine cells release some peptides and amines that signal via the vagus nerve to the brainstem, these substances elicit a range of reflexes to control digestion and food intake, nevertheless, they exert systemic anti-inflammatory effects [7]. It is possible that some of these anti-inflammatories may also impact the skin [8].

7.2.3 Immunological Interaction

Gut-skin communication occurs also through the immunological components that are present between the gut and the skin. One of the main functions of the immune system is Regulating the host's interaction with the microbiota, thereby the regions colonized by commensals, such as the skin and the GI tract, are covered with many immune cells. To achieve the host's homeostatic balance, the gut epithelial cell barrier, mucus layer, T cells, IgA, and dendritic cells (DCs) collectively shape the shield named 'mucosal firewall' The mucosal firewall prevents the translocation of commensal bacteria to the lymphoid tissues, limiting the inflammation of the gut and skin [9].

Recent studies have provided evidence that immune cell trafficking of the gut -that is derived from the skin- contributes to skin inflammation. Pathogenic immune cells can traffic from the skin to the gut, and the mechanisms of their migration appear to differ from those originating in the gut [10].

7.3 Skin Gut Axis and Microbiome

The microbiome refers to various microorganisms living inside human or animal bodies or on their skin. The microbiome also is the collective microbiota which is a term that usually refers to microorganisms such as bacteria, viruses, and fungi. There are two types of microbiota: commensal or nonpathogenic and pathogenic. There are thousands of microbiota present in humans, only several hundred are pathogenic, while the rest are commensal. Most microbiomes are commensal microorganisms. The microbiome is essential for immune system development and homeostasis whereas dysbiosis can lead to disrupted communication between the microbiome and the host, leading to an imbalance of the immune system [11].

The microbiota of the gut closely resembles that of the skin. Many studies have associated the inflammatory skin status with intestinal microbiota disorder. The intestinal microbiota affects the immunological function of the body and The immune system protects itself from external pathogenic bacteria. Once the intestinal microbiota is changed, the changed intestinal microbiota may lead to autoimmune and inflammation status not only in the intestines but also in faraway organs, including the skin. The gut–skin axis suggests a relationship in which the immune properties of the gut microbiota can also influence skin health [12].

Many studies have shown that pathogens and microbiota are associated with skin conditions, some of these pathogens are obvious and others are unknown until now. Nevertheless, it is difficult to determine if the altered skin microbiome is a cause or aftereffect of the skin disorder [3].

7.4 The Link Between Gut and Skin Diseases

Dysbiosis of the cutaneous and intestinal microbiome plays important roles in the pathophysiology of gut and skin-associated diseases, such as psoriasis, atopic dermatitis, acne vulgaris, rosacea, alopecia areata, and hidradenitis suppurativa [10] (Table 7.1).

7.4.1 Psoriasis

Psoriasis is an immune-mediated genetic skin disease affecting the skin and joints. The underlying Patho mechanisms involve a complex interaction between the innate and adaptive immune systems [17].

It is associated with improper activation of immune-mediated pathways that make the immune cells attack self-skin cells, resulting in increased levels of pro-inflammatory cytokines. Nevertheless, it is associated with two main important comorbidities Inflammatory bowel disease (IBD) and Crohn's disease [10].

Several studies provided more information regarding a correlation between the gut microbiome and skin health in psoriatic patients. For example, the genetic material of gut bacteria has been identified in plasma samples of patients with psoriasis [1, 13].

Moreover, Biomarkers of a damaged intestinal barrier have been observed among psoriasis patients [14].

Table 7.1 Link between gut and skin diseases

Disease/ condition	Skin gut axis evidence
Psoriasis	• The genetic material of gut bacteria has been identified in plasma samples of patients with psoriasis [1, 13]. • Biomarkers of a damaged intestinal barrier have been observed among psoriasis patients [14].
Acne vulgaris	• The adverse impact of a high-glycemic diet as well as common IBD comorbidity. • Several acne patients have also been found to develop low levels of stomach acid [14].
Atopic dermatitis	• Low intestinal microbial diversity during the first month of life was associated with subsequent atopic eczema [15].
Rosacea	• Exists with gastrointestinal comorbidities and confirmed a significant association in the occurrence of IBD, Not only but also coeliac disease, obesity, and insulin resistance [14]. • Diet and certain food items are known to trigger or worsen its symptoms [16].
Alopecia areata	• Many persons with AA also exhibit ulcerative colitis [9].
Hidradenitis suppurativa	• The adverse impact of a high-glycemic diet as well as common IBD comorbidity [14].

7.4.2 Atopic Dermatitis (Eczema)

Atopic dermatitis (AD), also known as (eczema), is a common chronic inflammatory skin condition characterized by pruritus [18].

Many studies suggest that gut microbial diversity facilitates AD. For example, Thomas R Abrahamsson et al. have shown that Low intestinal microbial diversity during the first month of life was associated with subsequent atopic eczema [15].

However, alteration of gut microbial composition alone cannot promote the development of AD. Interaction of specific microbes with the immune system, together with other external factors, such as diet, could better explain the pathogenesis of AD [9].

7.4.3 Acne Vulgaris

Acne is a chronic inflammatory disease of the pilosebaceous unit.

Several studies have indicated a correlation between gut dysbiosis with acne vulgaris [19].

The diet during acne vulgaris supports the existence of gut–skin axis. High-glycemic diet is a well-established aggravating factor in acne vulgaris and on the other hand Low-glycemic diet is associated with acne vulgaris improvement. Several acne patients have also been found to develop low levels of stomach acid. This allows colonic bacteria to migrate to the distal part of the small intestine, creating conditions for intestinal dysbiosis and growth of small intestinal bacteria, which can increase intestinal permeability and promote inflammation of the skin [14].

7.4.4 Rosacea

Rosacea is a common inflammatory cutaneous condition with a complex unknown etiopathogenesis till now. Diet and certain food items are known to trigger or worsen its symptoms [16].

Rosacea is reported to exist with gastrointestinal comorbidities and confirmed a significant association in the occurrence of IBD.

Not only but also coeliac disease, obesity, and insulin resistance [14].

7.4.5 Alopecia Areata (AA)

Alopecia areata (AA) is a common chronic autoimmune disease, that affects up to 2% of the general population. The exact pathobiology of AA is still unknown [20].

Literature data indicates that when compared with a healthy population, a high proportion of persons with AA also exhibit ulcerative colitis, indicating an association of the gut with AA [9].

7.4.6 Hidradenitis Suppurativa (HS)

Hidradenitis suppurative (HS) is a chronic inflammatory disease derived from the pilosebaceous unit in intertriginous areas, that affects approximately 1% of the general population [21].

HS and acne vulgaris have the same characteristic features related to the gut skin axis such as the adverse impact of high-glycemic diet as well as common IBD comorbidity. This suggests the possible role of gut dysbiosis in HS pathology [14].

7.5 Probiotic and Skin-Gut Axis

Probiotics are nonpathogenic living microbiota administered to enhance microbial balance [22]. In the last few years, significant progress has been made in understanding the composition of skin probiotics and how dysbiosis affects skin health. Topical and internal probiotics in the form of various dermatological formulations are vital for the treatment of skin conditions. By regulating skin health and gut–skin axis interactions, probiotics can be used as potential management tools to suppress and improve skin diseases in multiple ways, including decreasing oxidative stress, suppressing inflammatory responses, and keeping immune effects [12].

One of the most popular probiotics is kefir, It is an ancient probiotic food known to positively impact the general condition of the digestive system. The nutritional and microbial richness of kefir makes its application highly relevant within many sectors of healthcare. Although, the literature is still infrequent on the impact on the gut-skin relationship of a diet containing kefir, The existence of a relationship between the improvement in skin parameters and GI status after kefir taking was established. There are significant improvements in all skin outcomes [23, 24].

References

1. O'Neill CA, Monteleone G, McLaughlin JT, Paus R. The gut-skin axis in health and disease: a paradigm with therapeutic implications. BioEssays. 2016;38(11):1167–76.
2. Salem I, Ramser A, Isham N, Ghannoum MA. The gut microbiome as a major regulator of the gut-skin axis. Front Microbiol. 2018;9:1459.
3. De Pessemier B, Grine L, Debaere M, Maes A, Paetzold B, Callewaert C. Gut-skin axis: current knowledge of the interrelationship between microbial dysbiosis and skin conditions. Microorganisms. 2021;9(2):353.
4. Bradley WD, Zwingelstein C, Rondinone CM. The emerging role of the intestine in metabolic diseases. Arch Physiol Biochem. 2011;117(3):165–76.
5. Wood JM, Schallreuter KU. A plaidoyer for cutaneous enzymology: our view of some important unanswered questions on the contributions of selected key enzymes to epidermal homeostasis. Exp Dermatol. 2008;17(7):569–78.
6. Henke C, Beissner F. Illustrations of visceral referred pain. "Head-less" head's zones. Schmerz. 2011;25(2):132–6, 138.
7. Luyer MD, Greve JWM, Hadfoune M, Jacobs JA, Dejong CH, Buurman WA. Nutritional stimulation of cholecystokinin receptors inhibits inflammation via the vagus nerve. J Exp Med. 2005;202(8):1023–9.

8. Holzer P, Farzi A. Neuropeptides and the microbiota-gut-brain axis. Adv Exp Med Biol. 2014;817:195–219.
9. Mahmud MR, Akter S, Tamanna SK, Mazumder L, Esti IZ, Banerjee S, et al. Impact of gut microbiome on skin health: gut-skin axis observed through the lenses of therapeutics and skin diseases. Gut Microbes. 2022;14(1):2096995.
10. Zhang J, Yao Z. Immune cell trafficking: a novel perspective on the gut-skin axis. Inflamm Regen. 2024;44(1):21.
11. Sinha S, Lin G, Ferenczi K. The skin microbiome and the gut-skin axis. Clin Dermatol. 2021;39(5):829–39.
12. Gao T, Wang X, Li Y, Ren F. The role of probiotics in skin health and related gut-skin axis: a review. Nutrients. 2023;15(14):3123.
13. Ellis SR, Nguyen M, Vaughn AR, Notay M, Burney WA, Sandhu S, et al. The skin and gut microbiome and its role in common dermatologic conditions. Microorganisms. 2019;7(11):550.
14. Polkowska-Pruszyńska B, Gerkowicz A, Krasowska D. The gut microbiome alterations in allergic and inflammatory skin diseases—an update. J Eur Acad Dermatol Venereol. 2020;34(3):455–64.
15. Abrahamsson TR, Jakobsson HE, Andersson AF, Björkstén B, Engstrand L, Jenmalm MC. Low diversity of the gut microbiota in infants with atopic eczema. J Allergy Clin Immunol. 2012;129(2):434–40, 440.e1.
16. Searle T, Ali FR, Carolides S, Al-Niaimi F. Rosacea and diet: what is new in 2021? J Clin Aesthet Dermatol. 2021;14(12):49–54.
17. Kamiya K, Kishimoto M, Sugai J, Komine M, Ohtsuki M. Risk factors for the development of psoriasis. Int J Mol Sci. 2019;20(18):4347.
18. Bosma AL, Ascott A, Iskandar R, Farquhar K, Matthewman J, Langendam MW, et al. Classifying atopic dermatitis: a systematic review of phenotypes and associated characteristics. J Eur Acad Dermatol Venereol. 2022;36(6):807–19.
19. Williams HC, Dellavalle RP, Garner S. Acne vulgaris. Lancet. 2012;379(9813):361–72.
20. Zhou C, Li X, Wang C, Zhang J. Alopecia areata: an update on etiopathogenesis, diagnosis, and management. Clin Rev Allergy Immunol. 2021;61(3):403–23.
21. González-López MA. Hidradenitis suppurativa. Med Clin (Barc). 2024;162(4):182–9.
22. Williams NT. Probiotics. Am J Health Syst Pharm. 2010;67(6):449–58.
23. Alves E, Gregório J, Rijo P, Rosado C, Monteiro RL. Kefir and the gut-skin axis. Int J Environ Res Public Health. 2022;19(21):13791.
24. Alves E, Gregório J, Baby AR, Rijo P, Rodrigues LM, Rosado C. Homemade kefir consumption improves skin condition—a study conducted in healthy and atopic volunteers. Food Secur. 2021;10(11):2794.

The Effect of Different Diet Patterns in Acne Vulgaris

8

Jarjees Abduljabar Sulaiman and Esraa M. AlEdani

Contents

8.1 Acne with High Glycemic Index (GI) Diets

Foods like sugary snacks, refined grains, and processed foods that quickly raise blood sugar levels are included in a diet with a high glycemic index. It has been demonstrated that these foods set off a series of hormonal reactions, leading to an increase in insulin and insulin-like growth factor-1 (IGF-1) [1].

- **Insulin and IGF-1**: Higher insulin levels cause sebaceous glands to secrete more sebum, or oil, which is a major contributing factor to the development of acne. Furthermore, IGF-1 encourages the growth of keratinocytes, which are the cells that line hair follicles. This results in clogged pores and the development of acne lesions [2].
- **Clinical Findings:** Research has indicated that those with a diet high in high-GI foods are more likely to get acne than people with a low-GI diet. Low-GI foods

J. A. Sulaiman (✉)
University of Duhok, Duhok, Iraq

E. M. AlEdani
Basra Medical College, Basrah, Iraq

E. M. AlEdani, H. I. Maibach (eds.), *Nutrition and Acne Vulgaris*, Updates in Clinical Dermatology, https://doi.org/10.1007/978-3-031-83677-0_8

include veggies, whole grains, and legumes. They also assist to keep blood sugar levels steady and may lessen the severity of acne [3].

8.2 Western Diet

The Western diet is composed of large amounts of refined sugars, saturated fats, milk, diary product, while it is low in fruits, vegetables, vitamins, and minerals. FoxO1 is suppressed by the Western diet, which results in an increase in the activity of the majority of the transcription factors that are involved in the process of sebaceous lipogenesis. The upregulation of SREBP-1c not only increases the total amount of sebum produced, but it also alters the composition of the fatty acids found in sebum triglycerides by producing a pattern of fatty acids that are both proinflammatory and comedogenic. mTORC1 activation is enhanced by the saturated fatty acid palmitate and its lysosomal translocation, but it is inhibited by the ω3-fatty acid eicosapentaenoic acid (EPA), a main fatty acid found in fish oil. It is therefore possible that comedogenesis is promoted by sebum-derived free palmitate, which may activate the cell proliferation of acroinfundibular keratinocytes through palmitate-driven mTORC1 signaling. It seems that current acne is linked to the consumption of milk, sugary beverages, fatty foods, and sugary products. As a result, this could lend credence to the idea that adult acne is linked to the Western diet, which is heavy in meat, fat, and sugar [4].

8.3 Mediterranean Diet

The Mediterranean diet is primarily a plant-based diet that evolved and spread throughout the Mediterranean Basin before globalization had an impact on traditional dietary systems. The Mediterranean diet (MD) is based on the consumption of olive oil as the primary source of fat on a regular basis, as well as the consumption of a large quantity of fruits, vegetables, and grains. Additionally, the MD permits a moderate consumption of white meat, fish, and wine, while restricting the consumption of carbohydrates and red meat [5].

the severity of acne is not associated with consumption of the Mediterranean diet, while the Mediterranean diet is more play a protective role against the acne [5].

8.4 Plant-Based Diets and Acne Plant-Based Diets

Which emphasize the intake of whole grains, legumes, nuts, and fruits are generally linked to a decreased risk of acne [6].

- **Effects on Oxidative Stress and Inflammation**: These diets are high in antioxidants such vitamins A, C, and E, which help to lower inflammation and oxidative stress, two factors that contribute to the genesis of acne. They also include fiber, which lowers blood sugar and reduces the risk of insulin surges [6].

- **Low-Glycemic Nature:** The majority of foods derived from plants have a low glycemic index, which helps to lower IGF-1 levels and prevent insulin spikes [6].
- **Plant foods rich in omega-3 fatty acids** include walnuts, chia seeds, and flaxseeds. These fatty acids have anti-inflammatory qualities and may help lessen acne [6].

8.5 Dairy Consumption and Acne

Numerous studies have examined the relationship between eating dairy and acne, with varying degrees of success. Because dairy products include hormones and have the ability to increase IGF-1 levels, it is thought that they worsen acne, particularly skim milk [7].

- **Milk's Hormonal Content:** Milk naturally contains growth hormone and androgen precursors, which can raise blood levels of IGF-1 and insulin. These hormones are known to stimulate sebaceous glands and enhance keratinocyte growth, contributing to acne development [7].
- **Inflammatory Reaction:** There has been evidence linking certain dairy products, especially those that are processed or low-fat, to heightened inflammation. Acne vulgaris is largely caused by chronic inflammation. This is one of the reasons whole milk is thought to be less likely to cause acne than skim milk [7].
- **Evidence:** There appears to be individual diversity in the response to dairy consumption, since some observational studies have identified a positive correlation while others have reported weaker or no relationships between dairy consumption and acne. For example, yogurt and cheese don't seem to cause acne the same way that milk does; this could be because of the fermentation process [7].

8.6 Role of Specific Nutrients in Acne

Acne development and therapy are also linked to a number of certain nutrients that can be present in different dietary patterns:

- **Vitamin D:** A vitamin D deficiency has been associated with an increased risk of acne. Vitamin D possesses immunomodulatory and anti-inflammatory properties. Insufficient people may find that their acne clears up with supplements [8].
- **Zinc:** An important mineral, zinc affects inflammation and the immune system. Acne has been linked to zinc deficiency, and supplementation has been demonstrated to lessen acne severity, especially in inflammatory forms [8].
- **Probiotics:** Consuming fermented foods and probiotics as part of a diet that promotes gut health may help reduce acne. According to the gut-skin axis, inflammation and acne may be caused by dysbiosis, an imbalance in the gut microbiota, and symptoms may be mitigated by increasing gut health through diet [8].

References

1. Guertler A, Volsky A, Eijkenboom Q, Fiedler T, French LE, Reinholz M. Dietary patterns in acne and rosacea patients—a controlled study and comprehensive analysis. Nutrients. 2023;15(20):4405.
2. Melnik BC. Linking diet to acne metabolomics, inflammation, and comedogenesis: an update. Clin Cosmet Investig Dermatol. 2015;8:371–88. https://doi.org/10.2147/CCID.S69135.
3. Yasuda M, Tanaka Y, Kume S, Morita Y, Chin-Kanasaki M, Araki H, Isshiki K, Araki S, Koya D, Haneda M, Kashiwagi A, Maegawa H, Uzu T. Fatty acids are novel nutrient factors to regulate mTORC1 lysosomal localization and apoptosis in podocytes. Biochim Biophys Acta. 2014;1842(7):1097–108. https://doi.org/10.1016/j.bbadis.2014.04.001.
4. Penso L, Touvier M, Deschasaux M, Szabo de Edelenyi F, Hercberg S, Ezzedine K, Sbidian E. Association between adult acne and dietary behaviors: findings from the Nutrinet-Santé prospective cohort study. JAMA Dermatol. 2020;156(8):854–62. https://doi.org/10.1001/jamadermatol.2020.1602.
5. Trichopoulou A, Lagiou P. Healthy traditional Mediterranean diet: an expression of culture, history, and lifestyle. Nutr Rev. 1997;55(11 Pt 1):383–9. https://doi.org/10.1111/j.1753-4887.1997.tb01578.x.
6. Trichopoulou A, Martínez-González MA, Tong TY, Forouhi NG, Khandelwal S, Prabhakaran D, Mozaffarian D, de Lorgeril M. Definitions and potential health benefits of the Mediterranean diet: views from experts around the world. BMC Med. 2014;12:112. https://doi.org/10.1186/1741-7015-12-112.
7. Taha S, Shakhshir M, Zyoud SH. Acne Vulgaris and adherence to the mediterranean diet among university students: a case–control study. J Health Popul Nutr. 2024;43(1):41. https://doi.org/10.1186/s41043-024-00535-1.
8. Skroza N, Tolino E, Semyonov L, Proietti I, Bernardini N, Nicolucci F, La Viola G, Del Prete G, Saulle R, Potenza C, et al. Mediterranean diet and familial dysmetabolism as factors influencing the development of acne. Scand J Public Health. 2012;40(5):466–74. https://doi.org/10.1177/1403494812454235.

Correction to: Nutrition and Acne Vulgaris

Esraa M. AlEdani and Howard I. Maibach

Correction to:
E. M. AlEdani, H. I. Maibach (eds.), *Nutrition and Acne Vulgaris*, Updates in Clinical Dermatology, https://doi.org/10.1007/978-3-031-83677-0

This book was recently published. The following chapters have been corrected.

Chapter 2

The author affiliation was updated incorrectly and has been corrected as below in the revised publication.

Current Author Order
Esraa Mohammed AlEdani

Updated Author Order
Madona Pakkam, Esraa Mohammed AlEdani*

*Corresponding Author

Affiliation of Madona Pakkam
Department of Radiology, Mayo Clinic, Rochester, MN, USA

The updated version of these chapters can be found at
https://doi.org/10.1007/978-3-031-83677-0_2
https://doi.org/10.1007/978-3-031-83677-0_6

E. M. AlEdani, H. I. Maibach (eds.), *Nutrition and Acne Vulgaris*, Updates in Clinical Dermatology, https://doi.org/10.1007/978-3-031-83677-0_9

Chapter 6

The author affiliation was updated incorrectly and has been corrected as below in the revised publication.

Current Author Affiliation
A. S. Ghattas
Faculty of Medicine, Cairo University, Giza, Egypt

Department of Pharmacology and Toxicology, Faculty of Pharmacy, Tanta University, Tanta, Egypt

Updated Author Affiliation
A. S. Ghattas
Faculty of Medicine, Cairo University, Giza, Egypt

Index

E. M. AlEdani, H. I. Maibach (eds.), *Nutrition and Acne Vulgaris*, Updates in Clinical Dermatology, https://doi.org/10.1007/978-3-031-83677-0

GPSR Compliance

The European Union's (EU) General Product Safety Regulation (GPSR) is a set of rules that requires consumer products to be safe and our obligations to ensure this.

If you have any concerns about our products, you can contact us on ProductSafety@springernature.com

In case Publisher is established outside the EU, the EU authorized representative is:

Springer Nature Customer Service Center GmbH
Europaplatz 3
69115 Heidelberg, Germany

Batch number: 10732090

Printed by Printforce, the Netherlands